PAINTED
FACES

PAINTED FACES

A COLOURFUL HISTORY OF COSMETICS

SUSAN STEWART

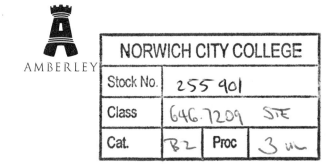

A work of considerable interest and extent might be written on the subject of cosmetics and the diversified modes of personal embellishment resorted to by various nations in different ages of the world. The singular and often dissimilar taste as which have influenced mankind in this respect would afford a volume no less amusing than instructive.

The Satirist, or The Censor of the Times (1843)

First published 2017

Amberley Publishing
The Hill, Stroud
Gloucestershire, GL5 4EP

www.amberley-books.com

Copyright © Susan Stewart, 2017

The right of Susan Stewart to be identified as the Author of this work has been asserted in accordance with the Copyrights, Designs and Patents Act 1988.

ISBN 978 1 4456 5399 0 (hardback)
ISBN 978 1 4456 5400 3 (ebook)

British Library Cataloguing in Publication Data.
A catalogue record for this book is available from the British Library.

Typesetting and Origination by Amberley Publishing.
Printed in the UK.

CONTENTS

I

INTRODUCTION:
MAKE-UP MATTERS

The *Oxford English Dictionary* defines a cosmetic as 'a preparation applied to the body, especially the face, to improve its appearance'. This broad definition encompasses eye make-up, hair dyes and face powders, lipsticks and rouges, foundations and creams, depilatories and deodorants. Trends in make-up emerge, disappear and re-emerge. Although some, like the popularity of rouge or blusher and the desire to preserve youth (through the use of face creams for example), never really go away, over the centuries there has been frequent shifting of emphasis as to how make-up should be worn; what was 'in fashion' if you like. In the past, however, fashion, as we shall discover, was rarely the only motivating factor. There were other, no less important motives behind the purchase, possession, application and the wearing of these products. While in today's world make-up is generally applied with the express intention of maximising the aesthetic appeal of the face and body – in particular, the female face and body – in the past, cosmetics were just as likely to be worn as visible markers of social status or religious expression, of gender, wealth, health and well being: that is to say, the meaning of make-up went well beyond mere decoration. Women and, at certain times in history, men have applied cosmetics to improve, alter, even to camouflage or disguise their appearance and have used cosmetics extensively as a visible clue to their health, wealth and social status.

Because of its wider significance, researching make-up, its uses, ingredients, its context and application, can provide clues not only to the nature and circumstance of the individual but can also help us to interpret the social, economic and political condition of society as a whole in any given period. That is to say, studying cosmetics can further our understanding of history. Here are a few examples of how this works. In Ancient Egypt, eye make-up was very important not only from the point of view of beauty but also for health and religious reasons: heavy make-up protected the eyes from heat and dust and was believed to guard against evil. Later on, the Romans valued elaborate make-up containers as symbols of individual wealth and status. In the medieval period, the church roundly condemned the use of cosmetics but by doing so, drew attention to contemporary interest in beauty. In the seventeenth century and into the first half of the eighteenth century, ostentatious hair pieces and wigs were *de rigueur* for men and women, an expression that was not about gender but about wealth and status. These fell out of fashion and favour following the political and social upheaval of the French Revolution because elaborate hairstyles smacked of the previous excesses of life at the French court; fancy hair styles were replaced by less showy arrangements that reflected the more sombre political and economic climate. At the end of the eighteenth century and into the early nineteenth century, skin care assumed greater significance as women, in particular, endeavoured to maintain their youthful looks and conceal any flaws that might suggest disease in order to acquire a husband. In the twentieth century, mass media such as cinema, television and ultimately the World Wide Web prompted rapid and almost impulsive changes in styles. Women copied the look and style of their favourite film or television stars. Make-up moved out of the privacy of the dressing room as women shared their beauty secrets on YouTube. Women openly applied their make-up on trains and buses and had it professionally applied at nail bars and brow-shaping services in open areas in shopping centres and department stores. Make-up had literally come out of the closet.

The Language of Cosmetics

The word 'cosmetic' was not, in fact, used until the beginning of the seventeenth century. Sir Francis Bacon (1561–1626), author, scientist and contemporary political figure, was the first to use the term. In the second book of his work *The Advancement of Learning,* published in 1605, Bacon defined cosmetic as 'the art of decoration'. The term make-up as a verbal phrase, meaning to put on make-up is used from 1808 but the noun 'make-up', referring to a cosmetic, does not become common parlance until 1886. Of course, cosmetics or make-up *per se* had been around for many centuries before the terms were actually applied. The Ancient Egyptians had their own individual words for different sorts of make-up: for example *mesdemet* was the ancient Egyptian word for eye make-up. In the classical world, the general term in Latin for beauty products was *medicamentum,* a word which included among its other meanings a medical remedy or a potion or enchantment. The form of the Latin word itself and the range of its meanings emphasised the close relationship between medicine and cosmetics in the ancient world and, to a greater or lesser degree, right up to the modern day. The Ancient Greek word equivalent to the Latin *medicamentum* was *kosmeticos* from which our English word 'cosmetic' derives. The etymology of *kosmeticos* implied a sense of order or harmony, the balance of the humors in Greek medicine – which in turn perhaps produced a pleasing and healthy appearance.

In the early modern period, cosmetics were referred to in general terms as 'paint', no doubt in part because the paint applied in the creation of a work of art was often the same substance used to adorn the human face and body. Specific products were not named. Instead, recipes were headed with vague titles, for example, 'a cream for the face' or simply 'toothpowder'. Sometimes recipes, or receipts as they were originally referred to, were grouped together with an indication as to their overall purpose. Under the heading 'how to make the hands fair and white' the reader might expect to find all the solutions known to the author that could achieve this effect, similarly with 'remedies to make the eyebrows black'. In the seventeenth and eighteenth centuries, many French words were used to refer to cosmetics whether as make-up in general, known as *fard*, or as brand name products, for example *Poudre D'amour, Serkis du serial* or *Eau de Lis*. This French terminology reflected the important influence of that country, and more specifically its capital Paris, on fashion and style. Names for individual products did not appear in any number until cosmetics became more of a commercial venture; initially the use of particular beauty products was attributed (and therefore at least tacitly endorsed) by high-status individuals and, in more recent history, cosmetic companies vied with each other to market and sell their products. Cosmetics give us an insight into what it was like to live in a particular era. Rouge, face creams and foundations, lipsticks, hair dyes, hair removers, teeth cleaners, eye make-up, deodorants and other cosmetic products have influenced and been influenced by contemporary attitudes, by people and by events, by increased knowledge and understanding (particularly in the fields of technology and medicine) and by trade and economics. They are a window into the past and can encapsulate the hopes and ideas of the future. In short, make-up matters.

Men and Make-up

Of course, a key function of make-up has always been to make the wearer more attractive to those who are doing the looking, that is, the viewer. Women have more often been the wearers, while men have done the looking. However, there are periods in history, especially in the seventeenth and eighteenth centuries, when men relied heavily on cosmetics to enhance and define their appearance and, more than that, to visually underline their importance in society. Even in times when make-up was not thought the done thing for men and when those who did wear cosmetics were roundly castigated for it, men have been remarkably keen to write about the subject of cosmetics. Much of the information we have about the use of cosmetics in the pre-modern world comes from men, who often criticised the use of these products. Their eagerness to do so can be interpreted as an indication of the popularity of beauty products but modern scholars argue that this enthusiasm for the subject is also borne from a fear of the power that female beauty can exert and, by association, a fear of the potential power of women within society itself; perhaps if we look at this on a more practical level, the worry of being duped into a marriage with a woman who is literally not what she seemed. This sense of the power of beauty may also be the reason why, through art and literature, men sought to set such a high standard for women to achieve in terms of appearance. Many women, of necessity, resorted to cosmetics in an effort to achieve the perfection set by the male-dominated societies in which they lived. As a result, descriptions of a woman adorning herself is an activity that often defines her gender but is viewed through the distorted mirror of the views and opinions expressed by men. Criticism of make-up expressed by men is common in the written record throughout history, even into the present day. Women as they are portrayed in works of art display perfection well beyond the average female member of society. No wonder these women resorted to cosmetics to try to reach this impossibly high standard. Societies as a whole, and men in particular, have struggled to come to terms with the artifice of cosmetics that attempts to replicate or even better natural beauty. Bias may on occasion distort the truth; the onus is on us to disentangle fact from fiction.

Women and Make-up

Although there are cosmetic recipes attributed to famous women in antiquity by male authors, there is really very little that we can be sure was written by women and that sheds light on how women viewed make-up or indeed the physical presentation of themselves. In the medieval period, the situation is much the same. Indeed the negative image that make-up acquired in the ancient world through rhetoric and satire is reinforced by the powerful influence of the early church. From the fifteenth into the sixteenth century, the period known as the Renaissance, women do begin to write down their own recipes and ideas in notebooks and even have these published. Important, well-known women in the pre-modern period are credited with using, recording, perhaps even inventing, various products and by so doing, either directly or indirectly, endorsing these – although this information was initially intended for private use within their own households.

Men continued to make their views known on this topic. However, while churchmen criticised cosmetics, diarists, doctors and others took a more pragmatic view, giving practical advice to women on how to make the best of their appearance. This guidance included advice on how to make and apply make-up. Early household management manuals gave instruction on how to care for one's skin, regarding this as essential knowledge that the woman, whether the mistress or servant attending her mistress, should have at her fingertips. The burgeoning popularity of ladies' magazines in the eighteenth and nineteenth centuries offered advice to women on how to look after their appearance. Newspapers carried discreet advertisements advising where to purchase various sorts of make-up and describing the benefits they claimed to impart. In the twentieth century, female emancipation influenced cosmetics and promoted self-expression through the use of make-up. Women were encouraged to look good (which might necessitate the use of beauty products) to boost morale, particularly during the Second World War. In the second half of the twentieth century, women followed the lead of the rich and famous in respect of appearance as feverish celebrity culture took hold. In the twenty-first century, some of the old ideas of the health benefits of cosmetics as well as modern ethical concerns about cosmetic testing on animals or recyclable packaging have come to the fore.

Setting the Limits

There is a vast amount of original material to sift through on the subject of cosmetics. Covering the ancient world, there are works of literature, as well as artefacts; some even with traces of the original products they contained still remaining. There are also paintings, sculptures and mosaics that even where they do not conclusively illustrate make-up *per se* depict the application of make-up. For the Medieval and the Renaissance periods we have cookery books, beauty manuals and so-called *Books of Secrets* as well as religious tracts, works of art and a few surviving artefacts. In the seventeenth, eighteenth and nineteenth centuries household books, pamphlets, newspaper advertisements, trade cards and magazines abound. In the twentieth and twenty-first centuries we find information about make-up in the media of photography, cinema and television. This amounts to a very long list of sources of information and a vast amount of useful material. However, it is impossible to include everything there is to say about this topic so, for the purposes of this book, it is necessary to set some boundaries, both practically and metaphorically. Firstly, I concentrate on the history of cosmetics in the western world with particular reference to Britain, France and Italy, countries that were often at the forefront of fashion and innovation in relation to make-up; the influence of America in the nineteenth and twentieth centuries is also covered. I include eastern ideas and cosmetic products that originated in the East only where these have in some way either influenced or been subsumed by the West. Secondly, the topic of perfumes is another vast area of research and warrants a book on its own. Therefore,

I confine myself to scented cosmetics and toilet waters rather than to any detailed study of perfumes. Thirdly, hair dyes, wigs and the cosmetics used to maintain or augment hairstyles are covered here but not the hairstyles themselves. Of course, fashions do change over time and the use of make-up is no exception. Even given the parameters outlined above, I have had to be selective. This book does not include everything there is to be said about cosmetics, and taking a broad brush approach, the text does not cover every nuance. I make no apologies for this. Instead this book is, I hope, a starting point for the general reader intended to highlight the importance of cosmetics as a topic and, I hope, generate further interest. I have chosen material where there is an interesting story to tell and where the relevance to the history of the period, or indeed to history in general, is clear. I look at some of the more intriguing people, stories and objects associated with cosmetics, as well as the ingredients and the finished products themselves. I do so in order to draw the attention of the reader to the topic as a means of learning about the past and indeed the impact of the past on the present. The reader may wish to refer to the glossary at the back of this book for some more scientific information about some of the words and terms that appear regularly throughout the main text. While the emphasis may mean that one side of the argument gets the upper hand against the other, and vice versa, here are some themes that are omnipresent throughout this book – the discourses of nature versus artifice, public and private, rich and poor, male and female, healthy and unhealthy, moral and immoral. All underpin the topic.

2

THE ANCIENT WORLD:
PRE-HISTORY – EGYPTIANS, GREEKS AND ROMANS

> Learn what treatment may enhance your face, girls,
> And the means by which you must preserve your looks
> Ovid, *On the Making up of the Face*

In the Beginning – Prehistoric Body Art

In the absence of the written word (that is, in the prehistoric era), we rely on objects, artwork and sometimes human remains for information. Our conclusions may be based more on logic and calculated interpretation than on any degree of certainty. This is as true when studying cosmetics as it is when focusing on any other aspect of the prehistoric past. It is, however, pretty clear from prehistoric paintings and artefacts that men and women did paint their bodies, and that we can interpret this as a practice that went beyond a desire simply for decoration or adornment. Body art was almost certainly a necessary element of participation in religious ritual. In time of conflict, decorating or tattooing the body in this way might quite literally be described as war paint; that is, make-up applied with the express purpose of creating a fearsome appearance to intimidate the enemy. Indeed historians and archaeologists studying prehistory believe the patterns and materials used in body art can indicate an individual's social status and the social group to which he or she belonged. Naturally occurring mineral pigments such as red or yellow ochre (earths containing iron oxide) were used in wall paintings but also to paint the surface of the human body. Powdered haematite, a sparkling mineral, was also applied on both the walls and on bodies – adding an aesthetically pleasing bit of showy glitter.

A male mummy of the ancient Chinchorro culture of Chile (dating from around 1800 BC) sports what appears to be a sort of tattooed 'moustache'. The well-preserved body of Ötzi, the Iceman, as he is often referred to, was found in an Alpine glacier along the Austrian-Italian border, where he had died around 3250 BC. His body is marked by no less than sixty-one tattoos. These were created by applying fireplace ash or soot to incisions all over the body. These are both early evidence of an inclination to adorn the body for the purposes of beautification, as well as, perhaps, to signify belonging to a particular social group. However, the marks on body of the Iceman are also believed to have served some therapeutic function. A number of the small line incisions are positioned in areas where the body would have been covered either by clothing or by hair. Otzi seems to have suffered from arthritis and some of the marks are cited at pressure points (for example the ankles and behind the knees) and may be evidence of an early treatment similar to acupuncture.

Combs and other tools used in personal care and grooming have been found preserved in bog graves. One of the Chinchorro mummies was buried with a cosmetic palette, a flat stone on which he or she would have ground up pigments for use in adorning the body. Shells are mentioned in classical literature being used to hold cosmetics but the remains of pigment have been found in shells much earlier than this. Spondylus shells were treasured for their attractive shape and ridged surface. Examples containing lepidocrocite (red quartz crystal), haematite (iron ore) and pyrite (fool's gold) have been found at sites in southern Spain associated with Neanderthal settlements. In south western Greece, a shaft tomb lay undisturbed for more than 3,500 years. When it was finally discovered in the twentieth century, archaeologists established that it belonged to a male warrior of the early Bronze Age. The grave contained around 1,400 objects, including a well-preserved mirror – showing attention to grooming was a concern for both Bronze Age men as well as women. Other warrior graves from prehistoric times have been found to contain razors and tweezers alongside their weapons, showing that these men took daily care of their bodies – controlling hair growth, which would have prevented disease.

The Bronze Age frescoes found at Akrotiri on the Aegean island of Thera (also known as Santorini) and buried by a volcanic eruption in 1627 BC offer us a unique insight into the early use of make-up. The frescoes appear to show women with their cheeks painted with rouge. Other than their cheeks, the women are pale skinned while the men in these frescos have a darker skin.

Women are also shown gathering saffron, an expensive spice valued among other things for its yellow dye. Saffron may have been used from an early date as a cosmetic, as part of cultic ritual or as a medical treatment; one fresco at Akrotiri shows a woman using saffron to heal her bleeding foot. Aromatics, like saffron, produced from earliest times, were used in cosmetic ointments and as perfumes as well as for their medicinal qualities. Beeswax, honey, olive oil and resin and orris root were all put to use in this way.

Ancient Egypt

In the Early Dynastic period (3100 BC–2686 BC), The Old Kingdom (2686 BC–2181 BC) and New Kingdom periods (1550 BC–712 BC) especially, there were many burials, first in pyramids and later in tombs cut into the rock, that demonstrate that The Egyptian pharaohs, other members of the Egyptian royal family, as well as their senior officials, were buried with objects that were considered to be central to their everyday earthly existence. The custom grew from the belief that the deceased would need these things when they passed into the next life. In Ancient Egyptian tombs, archaeologists have discovered many fine examples of objects used to store or to apply cosmetics including mirrors, hairpins, eye make-up containers and applicators, combs, spatulas and cosmetic pots – all made from a range of different materials including marble, alabaster, wood and reed. Some of the most well-known examples were discovered in the tomb of the boy king Tutankhamen, where archaeologist Howard Carter and his team found a number of alabaster jars, some of them very elaborate. As Ancient Egyptian tombs were sealed and therefore largely air tight, not only have cosmetic containers survived but so have traces of the scent of the aromatic ointments and liquids they contained, and the remains of the original contents are sometimes preserved too. Indeed, archaeologists have reported detecting the fleeting smell of some these often heavily aromatic products when first entering a sealed tomb. Sadly, however, any residual aroma escapes on the initial opening of a tomb and, of course, cannot be instantly bottled.

While many cosmetic containers and tools used to apply make-up have been found in the tombs of the pharaohs, in reality men and women, at all levels of Egyptian society, used oils and ointments to keep themselves clean, to cover up any unpleasant body odour, to improve their skin tone or simply adorn themselves, to take part in special occasions or religious ritual and even protect themselves from evil.

Ancient Egyptian make-up was predominantly red, green or black in colour. For the wealthy and important in society, there was also the option of the colour blue. Henna might be used as a natural yellow or red dye for the fingernails. Colours probably had some symbolic meaning in Ancient Egypt; for example, it is thought that red indicated fertility and that yellow meant god-like and eternal. However, while there were certainly messages in this early media, much of the real meaning of colour as the ancient Egyptians perceived it remains a mystery. Suffice to say, these colours were all extracted from naturally occurring rocks and gemstones. Green malachite, blue azurite, red cinnabar, yellow orpiment are all naturally occurring minerals. Lapis lazuli, a semi-precious stone, was ground down to produce an expensive deep blue powder for use as a cosmetic. All of these natural resources were pressed into service for the purposes of the adornment of both the male and female body.

Cosmetics and Medicine

In the written historical record there is really no distinction between cosmetics and medicines; make-up was, in effect, considered a branch of medicine at this time. Ancient Egyptian medical papyri include recipes for toothpastes and hair dyes alongside treatments for stomach disorders, swellings and headaches. In short, while cosmetics were undoubtedly used to beautify or make someone more attractive, the same mixtures were also used to protect or even to heal. The aging process was likened to a disease. Cosmetic oils and creams were applied to moisturize the skin and counteract the effects of aging, essential in combating the dry climate. Some of the moisturising ingredients the Ancient Egyptians used are familiar to us today; such as olive or almond oil, and beeswax. One Egyptian manuscript, entitled *The beginning of the book on how to make the old young*, makes it clear that the Ancient Egyptians, in common with people living in the twenty-first century and indeed all those who have lived in the centuries in between, valued the appearance of youth and were concerned to stave off dry skin and wrinkles, the visible signs of age.

Mirrors, Palettes and Containers

The Ancient Egyptians admired their appearance in mirrors of polished metal. These were highly valued objects and among an individual's most treasured personal possessions. Like other objects associated with the care of the body, mirrors were buried with the deceased in readiness for their use in the afterlife. Many were richly decorated. Palettes made of siltstone have also been found in Egyptian tombs. These were used as surfaces on which to prepare and grind up cosmetics, an eye make-up or perhaps a powder to tint one's cheeks. Cosmetic palettes with residue provide evidence of the use of a range of different make-up colours; red ochre used as rouge and green malachite or kohl (black) were ground up on a palette and mixed with a little liquid (water, rosewater or oil) for application as eye make-up, which became more ceremonial in purpose rather than for practical use.

The Egyptians kept their make-up in containers made from wood, alabaster, marble stone and ivory. The more important and the wealthier the individual was, the more elaborate the vessel was likely to be. A valuable pot or box was also an indication of the value of its contents. Containers that would be seen by others in the homes and palaces of the rich were as much an expression of the owner's personal status as they were a clue to their actual contents. One Ancient Egyptian make-up box on display in The British Museum dating from the New Kingdom time-period may once have belonged to Tutu, the wife of Ani, an important Egyptian official. The box is plain but made of good quality wood and contains a fine ivory comb, a pumice stone (for removing unwanted body hair) an eye make-up container, eye pencils (made of wood and ivory), a bronze mixing dish and three other containers (two made of alabaster and one of pottery). This is a functional quality piece, which aptly expresses the practicality of wearing make-up alongside the aesthetic and ideological ideas of beauty, wealth and status that were associated with body care at this time.

Ancient Manufacturing: Modern Analysis

In Ancient Egypt, the manufacture of beauty products often took place within royal palaces or at sites of great religious importance. Cosmetic production was strictly regulated. There was even an air of mystery preserved around the exact method of manufacture of some cosmetics and their actual composition; such was the value of both the ingredients in these cosmetic pastes, perfumes and ointments as well as the finished products themselves. Those people employed to work with the valuable aromatic resin frankincense were even searched on leaving their place of work to make sure they were not absconding with the product hidden anywhere on their person. With modern advances in science, it is now possible, using a relatively inexpensive technique known as Gas Chromatography-Mass Spectrometry, or GC-MS for short, to analyse small amounts of residue in order to find out what these beauty products were originally made of, without damaging their often equally precious containers. The Louvre in Paris owns about 500 Ancient Egyptian cosmetic containers and the cosmetics manufacturer L'Oreal has worked with the museum in an effort to find out what these once contained, using these new scientific methods of analysis. The results obtained show that many Ancient Egyptian cosmetics contained lead, which is dangerous not only to the skin but also, with continued use, to the proper functioning of the internal organs. Analysis of the remains also indicates that the Ancient Egyptians created subtly different powdered make-up by crushing the powder either very finely to make a dull or matt powder or by crushing the ingredients less finely to make larger crystals that reflected light and resulted in a shimmering finish.

Eye Make-up

There is little more obvious among cosmetics than the eye make-up worn by men and women depicted in the paintings on the walls of magnificent Ancient Egyptian buildings. Kohl, traditionally made from ground antimony or stibnite (a grey sulphide mineral) was used to create the almond shape around the eye that we are so familiar with in Ancient Egyptian art. This may also have had the effect of making the eyes look wider and more prominent as it contracted the eyelids helping to create the look that was much admired at the time. Take a look at the famous death mask of Tutankhamen and it is clear that he is wearing kohl. However, the boy king is far from unusual in this. Most Egyptians, not just the social elite, applied kohl – though wealthy Egyptians, both men and women, might also wear lapis lazuli alongside kohl on their eyes and eyelids. Alternatively they might use malachite, a powder made from copper that produced a bright and popular green shade. Green eye make-up was believed to promote fertility. The Ancient Egyptians also wore galena, a potentially dangerous copper and lead sulphide mix. In fact, Egyptian eye make-up presents us with a fine example of the three intertwined ideas that were associated with cosmetics in general at this time: that is, beauty, religion (or what we might term magic) and medicine. In the first place, kohl, made from antimony or lead sulphide, defined the distinctive ancient Egyptian shape of the eye creating the almond shape that was much appreciated from an aesthetic point of view. Secondly, the Ancient Egyptians believed that eye make-up reduced the risk of eye infections and even improved poor eyesight. Medical papyri tell us that kohl was prescribed as a treatment for eye disease. Thirdly, the heavily lined eye with its characteristic arrangement of heavy black lines and known as The Eye of Ra recalls the gods Horus, god of the sky and Ra, god of the sun, whom the Egyptians believed would protect the wearer against various diseases. They also believed that the cosmetic, and the symbolic design created with it, had the power to combat evil.

Ancient Egyptians stored their eye make-up in containers consisting either of a single tube or two tubes joined together. Where the container consisted of two tubes, the kohl powder was stored in one half of the container while a liquid (water or perhaps scented oil such as rose oil) was stored in the other. Having mixed the two together with a spoon or spatula on a small palette, one simply used a pin or stick to apply the make-up to both the upper and lower eyelids. In reality, kohl probably did give some protection from the sun and sand. Galena too may have antibacterial properties and repelled the flies that are always a problem in a hot climate. However, both substances (kohl and galena) also contained lead and were therefore potentially poisonous, even deadly. That is to say, alongside any initial protective benefits there was always the possibility that these cosmetics could, in the longer term, have the opposite effect and irritate the eyes rather than soothing and protecting them and cause other, even internal, damage.

Skin Care

The Ancient Egyptians applied ground alabaster (a soft white stone) mixed with salt or honey, milk and natron (a salt mixture locally available from dried lake beds) as a facial scrub and cleanser. Natron, also used in the mummification process to dry out the dead bodies, is known today for its effectiveness in removing dirt and grease, both as a household cleaner and as a body scrub. Beeswax, the substance with which the worker bees make the honeycomb, was applied all over the body as a moisturiser. This was also used on the lips to protect them from the harsh, arid conditions of the Egyptian desert. Face masks made of mud from the river Nile and alum (a white or colourless metallic compound) were believed to combat wrinkles. A more expensive combination of aromatic resins, namely frankincense and myrrh, mixed with animal fat, might also be used to moisturise the skin if you had the money to afford this treatment. The Ancient Egyptians do not appear to have worn much face powder, though they may have worn yellow ochre to tint their complexion just a little. The evidence for the use of lipstick in Ancient Egypt is rather scanty. However, the Egyptians probably did apply red ochre to colour both their lips and their cheeks and may have used red dye made from steamed, crushed and powdered beetles called lac, a red substance secreted by an insect of that name, to paint their lips as well. Body art or tattooing was popular among the Egyptian women in particular, just as it had been among earlier prehistoric people. However, just who had themselves tattooed, and exactly why they did so, is not clear. It may be that this was a fashion largely confined to lower-class women or possibly to those involved in the sex industry, including royal concubines. On the other hand, these markings may have a therapeutic or protective function, perhaps connected with childbirth and therefore been worn by women at all levels of society.

Hair

In terms of facial hair, the pharaohs favoured being clean-shaven but both the male and female rulers wore false beards to align themselves with the god Osiris. The Ancient Egyptians shaved their heads and wore wigs. Wig boxes have been found among the elaborate grave contents of the pyramids in the Valley of the Kings. While they wore these wigs in part to avoid lice and keep themselves free from other similar infestations, clearly this was not entirely successful as surviving examples of Ancient Egyptian wigs have been found to contain dead lice. The wigs themselves were moisturised and scented. Perfume cones made of beeswax combined with fragrant oils are often depicted in works of art. These were probably worn by members of the upper classes on ceremonial occasions. The wax cones are believed to have been up to 10 centimetres tall. In the heat, the wax melted and imparted the scent to the wearers' hair. The beeswax also kept the hair style in place. Unfortunately there are no surviving examples of these perfumed cones. Looking for traces of scented wax on surviving wigs would require some detective work that as far as I am aware has not yet been undertaken.

Although the Ancient Egyptians wore wigs, they also seem to have taken good care of their own hair, treating hair loss and colouring their hair to cover grey. A mixture of dried leaves and twigs of the henna plant might be applied to the hair to give it a reddish brown tint. The Ebers Papyrus, an early medical text dating from 1550 BC, so called because it was originally purchased, (as such artefacts could be in the nineteenth century), by one George Ebers, a German archaeologist, when visiting Luxor, recommends the following concoction to remedy grey hair: 'Donkey liver, leave in a pot until it is rotten. Cooked, put in lard. Rub in'. While the instruction is simple it is unlikely to have been effective. One thing we can be sure of is that the mixture would have had a very pungent odour. The Hearst Medical Papyrus dates to the first half of the second millennium BC and was named after Phoebe Hearst, a philanthropist in her own right and the mother of William Randolph Hearst, the famous newspaper publisher. The papyrus recommends a similar procedure but uses the by-product from a different animal: 'Cook a mouse, put in lard until it has rotted'. Again the method is reasonably simple, the likelihood of success remote and the smell abhorrent, at least to modern tastes.

Combating Body Odour and Bad Breath

Basic hygiene and make-up went hand in hand. Egyptian society, at all levels, strived to control unpleasant body odour. Strenuous efforts were made to keep the teeth clean. One Ancient Egyptian toothpaste recorded on papyrus reads as follows: 'A powder for white and perfect teeth made of rock salt, mint, and dried iris flower crushed pepper and mixed with natron'.

This would have been an effective mixture as it combines a breath freshener (mint and natron) with antiseptic and naturally abrasive ingredients including rock salt. Though potentially quite effective as toothpaste, if used too often this mixture might spoil the enamel on your teeth.

To avoid bad breath or halitosis, the Egyptians chewed herbs or leaf of natron to keep the breath fresh and cut down on tooth decay. Both men and women used body deodorisers. Low-paid workers in Ancient Egypt were routinely issued with a free supply of body oil for their daily use. No one wanted to work beside someone who smelled unpleasant. The Ebers Papyrus records the following treatment for body odour: 'A remedy to stop smells in a man or a woman: crushed carob pod is shaped into pellets and the body is anointed with it'. Certainly the carob seed pod does have a very strong aroma of its own which may well have masked body odours. Hair removal helped to control both body odour and the spread of lice. Arsenic compounds such as orpiment, a naturally occurring bright yellow mineral, was used to remove unwanted body hair. The Hearst Papyrus gives us the following hair removal remedy described as effective in 'removing hairs from any body parts': 'Boiled bones of the gbg bird, fly dirt, lard, sycamore milk, gum, a lump of salt. Warm. Apply.' We don't know what species of bird this was, but 'gbg' is what the Ancient Egyptians called it.

Cleopatra

The famous Queen Cleopatra was in fact the seventh Queen of Egypt of that name. She was anointed Queen at just seventeen, instantly becoming a woman of great power. Having had an affair with Julius Caesar, the most powerful man in Rome, she married his adversary Marc Antony in a bid to overthrow Julius Caesar's nephew Octavian. Ultimately she backed the losing side and, having been defeated, committed suicide. History says she used her beauty to increase her power and influence. Cleopatra was reputedly famous for trying to preserve her skin by bathing in asses' milk. Milk is easily absorbed by the skin making it soft, so

Cleopatra's milk baths might have worked as a beauty treatment. According to the Greek doctor Galen (AD 130–AD 210) who worked for the Roman emperor Trajan, Queen Cleopatra even wrote a book about cosmetics. Galen quotes her recipe for curing baldness, which involves an application of the crushed heads of mice or alternatively mouse droppings. Although Galen and indeed other authors of relatively early medical texts such as the later seventh century Paulus of Aegina claim that the Cleopatra who wrote about cosmetics and Queen Cleopatra were one and the same, recent research has concluded that this is unlikely. If the text quoted by Galen and others can be attributed to a woman called Cleopatra at all, this was probably another Cleopatra altogether. Aside from the anecdotal evidence of the queen's use of beauty products, and the attribution of actual recipes to her, there is, however, some proof in the archaeological record that she did have an interest in beauty products. The remains of a factory that made scented products including perfumes, perfumed oils and ointments has been excavated at Ein Gedi, an area on the western shores of The Dead Sea. The factory dates from the time that Cleopatra was known to be on the throne, and records show that the site was connected with her. Whether one believes or disbelieves the evidence that claims the queen's personal use and interest in beauty products it is certainly safe to say that Cleopatra, like other Ancient Egyptians, would have worn make-up not only for beautification but for hygiene and religious reasons.

Ancient Greece and Rome

'Beauty is heaven's gift' said the Roman poet Ovid, writing at the end of the first century BC. Certainly the images of the supposed occupants of heaven, that is the gods and goddesses of the Greco-Roman pantheon, as they are presented in art and in literature, set a very high standard for the ordinary or even the less ordinary mortals (that is, the social elite) to aspire to. Women in particular were under pressure to meet this high standard. Among the upper classes, feminine beauty helped secure a good marriage. For those women lower down the social scale, good looks could earn one a living especially as far as those working as prostitutes, call girls or those serving in the *popinae* or eating houses were concerned – as the latter frequently provided the same services as those overtly engaged in the sex trade.

Youth, or the appearance of youth, was an essential element of feminine beauty at this time. The perfect woman possessed a pale skin with just a hint of a blush, large dark eyes and a body that was neither too thin nor too fat. Real women ended up pursuing an imagined ideal. By the late fourth century BC, women were using a variety of cosmetics to look as good as the goddesses they saw depicted in wall paintings, vase paintings or mosaics, the idealised goddesses and semi-divine beings that possessed all the attributes of great beauty.

Sculptures, on the other hand, although they offer us some fine examples of what was perceived as the ideal body shape in the classical world, lack the colours with which these were once painted. This makes them a somewhat different proposition when it comes to looking for evidence of cosmetics. While there is little among the art work that definitively shows real women wearing make-up, the woman at her toilette is a common subject, particularly in funerary sculpture, but also in painting and mosaic. Men, on the other hand, are never portrayed in art associated with cosmetics.

In the literature that has survived from the classical era, Greek and Roman authors who are, to all intents and purposes exclusively male, have plenty to say on the matter. Most frowned upon women wearing too much make-up. The use of cosmetics by older women was considered particularly suspicious and deceitful. Women using make-up to deceive a man was a common theme in literature and was also probably a real concern. There was constant debate over which was superior, natural attractiveness or beauty achieved with the aid of cosmetics.

The opinions expressed by male authors on women wearing cosmetics depended to a considerable degree on the genre in which the reference appears, as well as the intended readership and indeed the purpose of the text itself. While women strived to improve their appearance, they were at the same time severely criticised for doing so. For example, satire condemns while drama mocks the overuse of cosmetics and perfumes by older women in order to appear young. Indeed, this is a stock theme in comedy. More factual works such as Pliny the Elder's *Natural Histories*, although not always correct, sets out to explain. Ovid in his poetry is perhaps rather the exception to the rule. He extols the benefits of make-up as part of the sophistication of city living. Medical texts, written more often than not in Greek, deal with the subject in a systematic manner, working from the head to the toes, often concentrating on information that would improve disfigurement resulting from disease, such as skin care and hair loss treatments.

Despite the rhetoric, in reality, cosmetics formed an integral part of the culture of the great civilisations of Greece and Rome whose peoples used a variety of aromatic herbs, plant roots, flowers, woods, fruit, seeds and gum resins for cosmetic purposes. While many beauty products were plant-based, they also used minerals such as red or yellow ochre, and animal products including fat (from swans, sheep, pigs and bears), dung (crocodile and bird droppings for example) and musk, a glandular secretion from animals such as deer or antelope.

In his *Oeconomicus*, or *Book on Household Management*, Xenophon, a Greek author writing in the fourth century BC, makes his fictitious character called Ischomachus describe how he trained his wife to manage their household effectively. In the course of the text, Ischomachus chastises his wife for wearing 'A great deal of white face powder so that she might appear paler than she was

... with plenty of rouge so that she might seem to have a rosier complexion than she had.' Greek women applied white lead as foundation and red ochre or the red plant dye alkanet to affect a healthy colour. Although in the Ancient Greek world, women spent much of their time inside the house and this seclusion would, no doubt, have helped maintain the desired pale complexion, sometimes a little extra help was required. This, as we see from the remarks Xenophon put into the mouth of Ischomachus, did not always meet with approval.

Greek men probably used cosmetic products for hygiene purposes, for example, to combat body odour or to keep their beards, when they were in vogue, in good order. Hair dyes and wigs were not worn by the Ancient Greeks other than by the actors on the stage but scented oils to control one's hair style were in general use. The Spartans, in particular, were known for their attention to their hair, which they combed repeatedly using oils to keep their locks glossy. They paid particular consideration to their hair in time of war as they saw their locks as symbolic of their strength. In the other major city state of Athens, Solon – an early law giver – restricted the use of hair oil among men, as he believed they were using this to excess; there was no such restriction placed on women's use of hair oil at this time.

Trading in the Classical World

The Greeks and Romans were keen and adventurous traders. Exotic materials used as cosmetics, or as ingredients in cosmetics, were imported to be sold in shops and in markets in and around the important cities. These might come in liquid, solid or powdered form and were probably stored in large vessels for the sea journey to the cities, where they were decanted into smaller vessels for sale and use. The Greeks seem to have understood how making packaging look attractive encouraged the customer to buy. It may have been possible by looking at the shape of the vessel that the Greeks could tell what they contained. However, there is evidence of the reuse of vessels for something other than their original contents and this muddles any identification that the historian or archaeologist may attempt. A better understanding of weather patterns, in particular with regard to the timing of the monsoon season, coupled with the expansion of the Roman Empire into Egypt and beyond, brought more and more exotic goods into the cities of the Roman Empire and especially into Rome itself. The Emperor Tiberius expressed his regret in respect of the amount of money that Rome was spending on these goods, which were often very expensive. 'How are we to deal with the particular articles of female vanity,' he is quoted as saying, '… which drains the empire of its wealth and sends in exchange for baubles the money of the commonwealth to foreign nations even the enemies of Rome.' By the beginning of the Roman Empire, it was an established criticism of women, in the literary evidence at least, that their desire for expenditure on and the use of cosmetics was not at all moderate and went well beyond what was economically, and socially, acceptable. It is hard to know just how much was being spent on make-up as we only have very patchy records as regards prices. There are records stating that one woman in Roman Palestine was some time in the first half of the first century AD spending 500 aurei (valuable gold coinage) a day on cosmetics. This seems more likely to be excessive rather than typical. Pliny the Elder in his *Natural Histories* gives prices, though it is likely that these prices were fairly variable in terms of time and from place to place. In addition, there were cheaper grades and alternatives to the most expensive luxury items; for example, there were several grades of nard, a pleasant smelling resin that was imported in large or small balls for use in skin cleansers and to promote hair growth, as well as for its perfume. Many luxury goods, including some cosmetics, were imported from far-off lands and despite their good trading links, the

Greeks and Romans did not always know where these products that they bought on the fringes of their territories were coming from. Instead, myths circulated, no doubt by word of mouth, but also in written text, that made these goods sound even more exotic; for example *balsamum*, an aromatic resin used as a hair ointment, was rumoured to come only from the king's gardens in Judea. While this often-invented exclusivity may have tempted buyers it also pushed up the price. *Balsamum* was an expensive product. Although we do know that when goods came from afar this inflated the price, there was scope for local and regional trade too, which due to lack of transport costs might be a little cheaper. Roses, for example, were grown for the cosmetic and perfume industry in the fertile lands of Paestum in southern Italy,.

Beauty products were sold almost door-to-door by iterant traders as well as at regular markets in the town forums. There were also fashionable shopping areas in Rome and other cities where goods like these could be purchased from premises displaying their wares with counters open to the street. Shops selling a specific range of goods, such as make-up or perfume, were often to be found grouped together in the same area. According to Ovid, there were wig shops near the temple of Hercules in the centre of Rome. In Capua, another great trading city in the south of Italy, there was an area known as the Seplasia that was devoted to perfume sellers. The Subura was a fashionable, if slightly decadent, area of the city of Rome where cosmetics and perfumes could be purchased. In fact cosmetics, through increased trade brought about by the expansion of the Roman Empire, became quite widely available. In short, in terms of cost and availability there was something for everyone and everyone used cosmetics.

Medicine and Make-up

Doctors were more often than not Greek and medical knowledge in the classical world was largely of Greek origin. Medical practice was based on the four humors or vital fluids – that is blood, phlegm, yellow bile and black bile. These fluids had to be correctly balanced in order to maintain good health. The condition of the skin and hair was considered a reliable outward sign of a person's state of inner health. Therefore it was very important to look good on the outside to indicate wellbeing on the inside.

Not only were cosmetics applied for the purpose of adornment, they also often doubled as medical treatments. For example, almond oil, a skin softener used as hand and body lotion then and now, was also a treatment for skin disorders. Rose oil, a popular ingredient in ancient perfumes and eye make-up, has anti inflammatory properties. This was understood by the Greeks and Romans who used it as an effective remedy for swellings. Galen left behind a recipe for cold cream that he is understood to have developed, initially at least, to heal any minor wounds sustained by the gladiators in the Coliseum. Cold cream is so called because when the cream is applied to the skin the water it contains evaporates, leaving a pleasant coolness. Galen's cream consisted of olive oil, beeswax, rose petals and water. Interestingly the recipe, largely in its original form, appeared in pharmaceutical reference books as late as the 1930s.

Roman Women

While there is much heavy rhetoric in Latin which indicates that cosmetics were the prerogative of the prostitute, closer examination of the wide variety of evidence attests to widespread use across all levels of society. In the first century AD, the Stoic philosopher Epictetus tells us that young women were aware of advantages of applying a little powder and paint. He notes that young girls begin wearing make-up once they are fourteen to order to find a good husband. By the time of the Roman Empire, we have a very clear idea about what contemporary society thought a beautiful woman should look like. Roman artists and writers described Venus, the goddess of love and beauty, possessed of a porcelain pale skin, blonde hair and large dark eyes. Real Roman women wanted to look just like her. This meant looking as if you had not been outside in the hot sun even if you had. Well-to-do Roman ladies were somewhat freer to come and go from their homes than their Greek counterparts had been. Though these women did not work, they liked to go out to shop and to visit their friends, as well as attend festivals, games and other public events. The hot Mediterranean weather made it difficult to maintain a pale complexion without using cosmetics, though these women might also have sought the protection of a veil or even an umbrella. Women who worked in bars or as prostitutes to earn a living, as well as women who helped in their husbands' shops standing at an open counter with little protection from the sun, would have had to work harder to achieve the desired pale complexion.

Did Roman Men Use Cosmetics?

The answer is yes, they did. However, they did not get a very good press if they did so. Although men applying or wearing make-up is never subject matter in art, classical texts do refer to men as well as women wearing make-up. These references are always critical, declaring men who used make-up were too interested in their appearance and, as a result, unsuited to public life in the senate, law courts or elsewhere. Famously, the hideaway of the disreputable Catiline and his co-conspirators who plotted against the government in 63 BC was discovered because the strong smell of the perfumed ointments they were wearing gave them away. The satirist Juvenal accurately observes a male transvestite applying eye make-up and likens him unfavourably to the Emperor Otho admiring his appearance with a mirror in his hand. Although men were criticised for wearing make-up, they were required to follow basic hygiene practices. This would have involved the use of some cosmetic products and utensils; for example, removing hair from their armpits, perhaps with tweezers, to avoid infestations of lice, and keeping their breath fresh, no easy task when garlic and sour wine were so much part of their diet, by chewing spiced pastilles or leaves.

Roman Baths

In reality, both women and men used cosmetics to help keep their bodies clean, just as the Ancient Egyptians and Greeks had done before them. Soap had not yet been invented so the ancient Romans scraped the dirt from their bodies using oil and a strigil, a tool with a curved blade. Oil could be brought to the public baths in a globular shaped bottle or *alabastron*. Powders, similar to the dusting powders we might use after a bath today, were sprinkled all over the body, perhaps even over one's clothes, to make them smell pleasant. Hair pins which became stuck in the drains at public bath sites (for example, such as those found at the Roman baths at Caerleon in Wales) are common finds and indicate that the presence of women at the public baths was nothing unusual. Though claims have been made by earlier historians for the existence of beauty parlours at the baths these are, to date, unsubstantiated as no archaeological evidence for such facilities has been found. However Seneca, the philosopher, playwright and advisor to the Emperor Nero, complains about the noise of men shouting while having their underarm hair plucked out at the baths near his house so we can be sure that this was a service offered to men at the public baths.

The Toilette

Varro, a Roman scholar writing in the second century BC, describes the objects that belong to a woman's toilette set in rather vague terms as anything intended to 'beautify a woman'. In fact, mirrors, mixing palettes, spoons and spatulas, as well as boxes, jars and other sorts of containers, are among the objects associated with the toilette. Mirrors made of polished metal were precious possessions. Glass mirrors do not make an appearance before the third century AD. It is interesting to surmise that the image reflected by means of a mirror of polished metal was probably not very clear. If the reflection was of a poor quality, then a lady might have to rely on her female relatives or friends, or perhaps even her servants, for an accurate opinion on her looks. One can imagine that these opinions might not always be impartial.

Palettes similar to those that belonged to the Ancient Egyptian were used for mixing. Liquids were stored in glass bottles. Some of these glass containers had a narrow neck, which allowed the ingredients to be used drop by drop; the small test-tube shape container was very common. Others containers were for single use. For example, bird-shaped vessels are found in the North of Italy. It appears that the bird's tail was snapped off and the contents used all at once. Boxes made of a dense material such as onyx or alabaster were popular, as these helped preserve the precious scent of the cosmetic for longer. Vessels could be reused and refilled, not always with the contents they originally contained. Men and women used basic cosmetic tools such as tweezers and nail cleaners and often wore these suspended from a chatelaine or elaborate hook attached to a belt on their clothing. These simple practical everyday tools are found across the classical world in the remains of private houses, at the public baths and in military camps. Double sided combs with two different sets of teeth are also found regularly when excavating at Roman military sites. These are small enough to fit in to the palm of the hand and might have been used not only to delouse the hair and comb it through but also to hold it in place. Tongs, heated in the fire, were used to curl hair. The tools for mixing and applying cosmetics were kept together in a box called variously *castellum*, *myrothecium* or *narthecium*. The box could be transported from room to room in the Roman house or even to the public baths as required.

Women undertook the actual process of putting on their make-up in private, away from the eyes of men. The poet Ovid insists: 'Why should I know what makes your skin so white? Keep your door shut and don't let me see the work before it is finished'. Often only the servants were present, barely regarded as people as they had no real status of their own. Although in real life it was best etiquette for the doors to be closed, in drama the toilette scene appears in the somewhat formulaic Roman comedy in a public setting in more ways than one, that is, the entire action in all Roman comedy, including any toilette scenes, takes place outside in the street. Plautus' play the *Mostellaria* or *Haunted House* is a particularly good example of this. The young maiden is advised on her make-up by a crone while the male lover watches from the wings, as it were, and comments on the action. This *al fresco* presentation of what was considered a very private activity may well have been part of the humour of the play. It is testament to the Romans' familiarity with the toilette as part of everyday routine that they could afford to make a joke out of it, knowing that everyone in the audience would understand.

Wealthy Women

Roman ladies who belonged to the social elite had a large number of servants who were highly trained in the art of putting on make-up. The toilette is a common motif on funerary reliefs commemorating the deceased in a task associated with everyday life. Maidservants in paintings and sculptures such as the Neumagen relief may seem to us to look at each other anxiously as they carry out their tasks; and well they might. Roman authors tell us that if the mistress's face was blotchy or her hair out of place then these girls could be whipped, beaten and even stabbed with hair pins as the Satirist Juvenal describes:

> The wretched Psecas for the whip prepared
> with locks dishevelled and with shoulders bared
> Attempts her hair: fire flashes from her eyes
> 'Strumpet why is this curl so high?' She cries.

Instantly the lash without remorse is plied
and the blood stains her bosom back and side.

Not all mistresses treated their servants in this way but enough of them did for the poet Ovid, whose view of make-up is almost always a positive one, to express his disapproval of this sort of behaviour. He says, 'I detest her who tears the face of her attendants with her nails and who seizing the hairpin pierces her arms.' The wealthy Romans relied on their slaves, whom they kept in large numbers. They lived in fear of a slave revolt so no doubt some high class women did take to exercising their authority in this way to ensure their slaves were kept in their place. The cruel treatment of slaves is not depicted in classical art. Instead the number of servant girls shown, for example, in the Neumagen relief, and the size of the mirror in which the seated subject admires her reflection, are intended to convey the wealth and high social status of the mistress.

In the wealthiest households each individual servant might have a particular job to do, for example, carrying the box of cosmetics, applying scented hair oil or removing unwanted body hair. The hairdresser or *ornatrix* may have been the chief domestic servant for ladies, in charge of the other maidservants attending the lady of the house. Often a favourite, the legal codex compiled by the Emperor Justinian (482–565) states that a period of three months' training was required for this job.

In classical literature women were often accused of spending far too much time putting on their make-up. However, this may have been very necessary. The weather was a big problem. Cosmetics used in the classical period were not waterproof. If it rained, make-up ran down the faces of those wearing it. Also if the sun was too hot, the make-up simply dried up. Lots of time was spent repairing make-up and reapplying it over a day, especially after a trip outside on a rainy day or maybe a visit to the baths.

Working Women

While working women would not have had access to the more expensive cosmetics there were plenty of cheap alternatives. Those who worked as call girls serving perhaps one or two clients might obtain some more luxurious products by way of gifts from that client or clients. Poorer prostitutes who worked in the public brothels, inns in the streets, and even graveyards, relied on cheaper options to try to preserve their attractiveness. After all, their appearance was their stock-in-trade upon which they depended for their livelihood because there was no state aid. Shop signs showing female assistants have survived but give us no concrete information about the use of cosmetics by this sector of society. It is worth noting that the products or the ingredients to make cosmetics these women could afford were certainly available; indeed, some of these women might even have been selling them. However, for women working in shops or helping to run small businesses, the time needed to apply and re-apply (many were working outdoors) was probably in very short supply. These women were not ladies of leisure like their wealthy counterparts.

Eye Make-up

Large dark eyes with eyebrows that met across the bridge of the nose were considered fashionable and attractive. Pliny the Elder, in his wide ranging encyclopaedia *The Natural Histories,* says that he has heard that women fill the natural gap between their eyebrows with crushed flies. His choice of words suggest even he does not believe this. It is certainly hard to see how this would have worked. However, a mixture of soot and ashes, combined with saffron or charred rose petals to make the whole concoction smell pleasant, was applied carefully around the eyes to accentuate them, help make them look larger and, as a result, more beautiful. Powdered eye make-up made from kohl or antimony sulphide was used for blackening brows and lashes. Again, this could make the eyes look larger in contrast to the amount of the eyelid that remained visible. Eyelashes could be dyed. Pliny the Elder maintains than some women had their eyelashes dyed as part of their daily routine. While his remarks are intended, no doubt, to suggest the excessive lengths women would go to as far as their appearance was concerned, the daily application of eyelash dye also reminds us that many of the dyes used in the ancient world were not fast and would soon have become faded, worn or just washed off. While some cosmetics or their ingredients were undoubtedly expensive, others such as ash or soot were cheap and easily obtainable; the Roman oil lamps that lit the brothels and elsewhere were one obvious source.

Hair Dyes and Wigs

If, like Julia (30BC–AD14) the daughter of the Emperor Augustus, you had begun to ask your maid to pluck out your grey hairs, then it was time to try a hair dye. Hair dyes came in a variety of shades. Venus-blonde was very popular though according to the Greek playwright Menander (342–291BC), 'no chaste women ought to make her hair yellow'. Such criticism probably arose from the fact that blonde was not the predominant hair colour of the women or men living in the Mediterranean basin. Those who had blonde hair were more likely to be slaves imported from other countries such as Germany where blonde hair was far more common. However, both the Greeks and Romans appreciated the unusual and over the centuries, blonde became a popular shade. To get that blonde-babe look, saffron – the yellow dye that comes from the crocus flower – was applied to the hair. Alternatively, a lady could spend some time sitting in the sun to achieve a bleached effect, presumably covering her face at the same time to prevent that undesirable sunburn or those wrinkles. Although blonde hair was much admired, it was not the only shade that was appreciated. Dark hair was also deemed attractive. The poet Ovid clearly thinks highly of the striking contrast of raven black hair next to pale skin, which he describes the following lines: 'Black hair on snow white shoulders reminds of Leda raven locks'. Leda was a beautiful maiden seduced by the god Zeus while transformed into a swan. The poet reminds us that in the Greco-Roman pantheon not all divine beings or indeed those associated with the gods and admired for their beauty are described as having blonde hair. Dyes that coloured the hair black might be effective in covering grey and the signs of aging. Crushed elderberries dyed hair black. As the poor man's diet consisted of seeds and fruit, elderberries were probably not only cheap and affordable but also widely available. A dye made from leeches steeped in vinegar for forty days was also used to colour hair black in what was a lengthier and more expensive procedure. There were red hair dyes on the market too. Walnut oil served a double function. This was used to dye cloth and to dye hair red. The empress Julia Domna (AD 170–AD 217) a patron of the doctor Galen, not only relied on him for medical treatment but also encouraged him to include hair dyes in his writings. Clearly this was something in which she and the other ladies at court had an interest.

The trouble with hair dyes in ancient times was that they were often not very good for the hair. In fact, they frequently caused hair loss. However, there were products available that purported to counteract this and prevent one from going bald. For example, a mixture of bear's grease and goat's ashes could be applied to the bald patch. Another concoction of animal fat or myrrh with a resin from the rock rose from southern Arabia was thought to be effective against hair loss and even encourage hair growth.

If hair loss cures or hair growth products didn't work, and it is difficult to see how any of these concoctions could, it was time to buy a wig. When the Romans conquered the Germans, they shaved off their blonde hair to make fashionable wigs for their own wives and girlfriends. Although some men wore wigs, they hoped no one would notice as this was considered vain and a slight on one's character. The historian Suetonius, in his *Lives of the Caesars*, notes that the emperor Otho: 'By reason of the thinness of his hair of his locks wore a wig so closely fashioned and fitted to his head that no one could distinguish it.' He adds that this was not in keeping with the emperor's exalted status. Suetonius also remarks upon Julius Caesar's lack of hair and mocks him for wearing a wig. Although baldness in a man in the classical world could help to give the impression that he was a man of some seniority and therefore power, the bald man was also a well-known character from Roman comedy and someone who got lots of laughs. In literature, the meaning baldness depends on the context. In reality, men then – just like men today – didn't really appreciate losing their hair.

Unlike men who tended to wear their wigs discreetly, women who wore wigs often did so to get noticed. The statues of Severan empress Julia Domna, her sister Julia Moesia and other female relatives even had detachable hair so that their hair styles could be changed to whatever was in fashion at the time. On the other hand, the wrong choice of wig in the wrong place could cast aspersions on the morality of the woman in question. The empress Messalina, wife of the Emperor Claudius was much maligned for her excess. Juvenal describes her as donning a blonde curly wig to lead a debauched life as a common prostitute during the night. The colour and the style of the wig are meant to tell the story in themselves.

Foundation and Face Powder

Writers in the classical world compared the perfect complexion to elements of the natural world. The elegiac poet Propertius waxes lyrical on this theme. He says: 'Lilies are no whiter than my mistress. Picture Maeotian snow vying with Spain's vermillion and rose petals floating on pure milk'. The effect women in these times set out to attain was certainly not an easy one to achieve. The colours were subtle. The products applied were not always easy to use and, being harsh, could cause long-term damage that could only be covered up with yet more often harmful make-up. Despite the dangers, to help them keep that pale and interesting look, women used a poisonous white powder made from lead known as *cerussa* in Latin or in Greek *psimithion*. The preparation of this white lead is described in detail by Pliny the Elder and involved steeping lumps of lead in vinegar over a period of days to produce a fine whiter powder. Human bones dug up on archaeological sites dating from the Roman period often have a high lead content. However, we should not make too much of this in respect of the dangers of cosmetics. While the lead women in particular applied to their faces may have been a contributory factor, but the ingesting of lead through the lead pipes and the fact lead was even added, as a preservative, to the wine the Romans were drinking probably made a far more significant contribution to these very high levels. Among the Greeks and Romans, white lead was known to be poisonous. The Greek poet and physician Nicander writing in the second century BC gives us our earliest detailed, indeed graphic, description of the effects of white lead:

> This fluid astringes and causes grave ills,
> The mouth it inflames and makes cold from within,
> The gums dry and wrinkled and parched like the skin,
> The rough tongue feels harsher the neck muscles grip,
> He soon cannot swallow,
> Foam runs from his lip,
> A feeble cough tries in vain to expel
> He belches so much and his belly does swell,
> His sluggish eyes sway then he totters to bed,
> Fantastic forms flit now in front of his eyes,

While deep from his breast there soon issued sad cries,
Meanwhile there comes, stuporous chill,
His feeble limbs droop and all motion is still.

However just as we are aware of the dangers of some of our own habits (for example, smoking), the knowledge of these dangers did not stop the use of white lead. In fact, despite the alarming effects described by Nicander and others, the dangers of white lead would not be heeded and acted upon for centuries to come. Thankfully, there were a few safer alternatives to the application of white lead available to the Greeks and Romans. These included kaolin or china clay. Crocodile dung, which is white, could also be used to make one's face look pale – safer perhaps, but distinctly unpleasant.

A delicately flushed cheek, that is a natural blush, was deemed attractive, very feminine and an indication of good morals. Ovid, who was much in favour of make-up anyway, confessed to favouring the artificial version of the blush over which women could have some control.

Mulberry juice and left-over red wine could be used to tint the cheeks rose red. The mineral cinnabar was also applied to achieve this effect. The ancients believed red cinnabar to be the blood of the basilisk, the mythical king of the serpents and a creature well-known to *Harry Potter* fans. Imported from Spain and India, this was another highly dangerous cosmetic.

Anti-Wrinkle Creams

We know that Greeks and Romans believed beauty to be synonymous with youth. The poet Juvenal even went so far as to maintain that husbands would no longer love their wives when they grew older unless they avoided the visible signs of old age and kept their youthful attractiveness:

When you get to the root of it, what he loves isn't his wife but merely her face. When the first wrinkles appear, when her skin goes dry and slack when her teeth begin to blacken, when her eyes turn lustreless, then 'pack your bags' his steward will tell her.

Given the fact that Juvenal's verse is satirical, his statement is no doubt an exaggeration. However, the plethora of anti-aging creams on the market, particularly at the time of empire, are an indication that there was considerable interest in preventing wrinkles, even if we cannot say that these women necessarily feared the collapse of their marriage because of their failure to appear young and therefore beautiful. There is little or nothing to suggest that men used anti-wrinkle creams. Of the cosmetics on the market, swan's fat was thought to be one of the most effective though duck's, bear's and lion's fat was also used. It is tempting to believe that some of these animal fats might have been a by-product of the sport at the Colisseum, although there is no direct evidence for such a connection. Almond oil, still a popular moisturiser today, was applied to combat the signs of aging too. Stretch marks or wrinkles resulting from childbirth were smoothed away with a cosmetic made from beans ground down into flour. A cream made from the grease extracted from unwashed sheep or goats' wool, was a popular choice. However this is a cosmetic that the poet Ovid seems to dislike; he complains bitterly about its unpleasant smell. Our modern equivalent of the cosmetic Ovid describes is lanolin, a mixture of wool-fat and water, now used in everything from eyeliners to skin care products.

Archaeologists excavating the site of a Roman temple in Tabard Square London in 2003 uncovered a small tub of cosmetic cream still bearing the finger marks where the last person to use it had scooped out its contents. When the mixture was analysed it was found to consist mainly of animal fat with tin added as a preservative. The cream was also found to contain starch, obtained by treating roots or grains with boiling water. The presence of starch means that the cream would turn to fine powder on contact with the skin. Starch is still used to create foundations that give a matt powdered effect. The small container (made of tin) and its contents date from the second century AD and show that this sort of product, an anti aging cream that is sophisticated in its production, was available even in Britain, a remote outpost of the Roman Empire.

There is an earlier and less publicised example of an ointment pot with residue. This belonged to a high-status Etruscan woman (the Etruscans were a wealthy Italian civilisation that flourished from the eighth to the third century BC) called Thania Plecunia and was discovered in Chusi in Tuscany in 2005. The urn-shaped box not only contained tools but also included a pot of scented ointment which, despite lacking a lid, had survived almost intact due to favourable conditions. The mixture contained pine resin and mastic resin as well as Myrobalan oil more commonly called Moringa oil today. Archaeologists have concluded that the mixture was imported, already manufactured, from Egypt.

Face Packs and Body Lotions

Women followed their favourite gladiators, an early form of celebrity culture or hero worship. The sweat from the fighters was collected to be used as a body lotion. Bathing in asses' milk to whiten and soften the skin was also popular and had a long tradition going back to Queen Cleopatra. Pliny the Elder adds that some women bathed in milk seven times a day. The number seven had special meaning, adding an element of magic to this procedure and perhaps encouraged belief in the efficacy of the product. Poppaea Sabina, who married the Emperor Nero, becoming empress in AD 62, was famed for her great beauty and her attention to the care of her person. She was reputed to bathe in the fresh milk of five hundred asses every day very much in the tradition of the famous Egyptian queen. Poppaea also gave her name to a sticky bread-based face pack for use at night to whiten and smooth the skin and prevent spots – perhaps an early example of product endorsement by the rich and famous.

The poet Ovid wrote a poem entitled the *Medicamina Faciei Femineae* (*On the making up of the face*) of which, unfortunately, only 100 lines have survived. Here, as well as in his other works, Ovid writes consistently in favour of using cosmetics, believing them to be a necessary part of life in a sophisticated urban setting. The *Medicamina* describes various face packs which, according to the poet, would make a woman's face 'smoother than her mirror'. Plant grains including barley and lupin seeds mixed with wax were used to remove dead skin. In fact, all the surviving recipes in this short piece contain a strong exfoliating element in the form of crushed beans or lupin seeds and were mixed with wine and other liquids such as barley water. Here is one of these recipes:

Come learn from me how to impart a dazzling whiteness to your skin. Strip of its straw and husk the barley which our vessels bring to our shores from the fields of Libya. Take two pounds of peeled barley and an equal quantity of vetches moistened with ten eggs. Dry the mixture in the air, and let the whole be ground beneath the mill-stone worked by the patient ass. Pound the first horns that drop from the head of a lusty stag. Of this take one-sixth of a pound. Crush and pound the whole to a fine powder, and pass through a deep sieve. Add twelve narcissus bulbs which have been skinned, and pound the whole together vigorously in a marble mortar. There should also be added two ounces of gum and Tuscan spelt, and nine times as much honey. Any woman who smears her face with this cosmetic will make it brighter than her mirror.

The ingredients in the main are natural and have potential. Honey, plant grains and egg, for example, are not unknown as ingredients in modern cosmetics. The reader may also notice the large quantities of the individual ingredients. Either the mixture could be easily stored and kept over a long period or this was a supply for a number of women either living in a household or in some way connected with each other. There is much that we can read into this alongside a regret that more of the work did not survive. Suffice to say, dismissed as a piece of writing of inconsequential value for many years, the importance of this text is only just coming into its own.

Hair Removal

Both Greek and Roman men and women removed underarm hair with tweezers. The Greeks also singed their unwanted hair to get rid of it. The Romans either plucked out the hairs individually or used caustic products that risked removing the top layer of the skin with the unwanted hair if left on the skin for any length of time – mixtures composed of quicklime or arsenic for example. Both civilisations used various depilatories made from some very strange ingredients: owls' blood or a mixture of beaver oil and honey, for example. It seems very unlikely that these treatments would have been effective as hair removers. Indeed Pliny the Elder, while quoting these recipes, indicates that the hair should be removed first. It is difficult to understand this other than by interpreting some of these mixtures not as hair removal procedures *per se* but as substances that would prevent the hairs from growing again once they had been plucked out or burnt off. Hair could also be rubbed off using naturally abrasive pumice stone. Besides the removal of underarm hair, the practices of men and women differed. Women's bodies were expected to be devoid of all hair while men did no more than remove the hair from under their arms.

Teeth

In the classical world bad teeth including black or marked teeth was a sign of poverty. Lack of teeth was clear evidence of aging, a process, you will recall, that was treated very much like a disease. Both black teeth and lack of teeth could also be taken as a sign of general ill health. Therefore keeping one's teeth clean and one's breath fresh was essential for any respectable citizen. This was not necessarily an easy task given the wine and spicy food that was part of the contemporary diet. Tooth powders made from pumice stone or ground animal bones were used to clean the teeth. Leaves from the laurel tree could be chewed to freshen the breath and one perfumer named Cosmus, according to the Roman epigrammatist Martial (AD 40–AD 140), sold pastilles for this purpose. Some analysis of the teeth from bodies found at Pompeii and Herculaneum, preserved under the ashes spewed out by the volcanic eruption of Mount Vesuvius in AD 79, has been carried out. As one would probably expect, the findings from person to person vary considerably – different people, varying status, different diets and hygiene practices are all factors that could have contributed to this variation.

Tattoo Removal

Roman slaves were branded or tattooed but under Roman law, slaves could be freed by their masters. It was quite possible that a Roman freedman (or woman) as he (or she) was known, although ineligible for public office could become a very wealthy member of society. Almost inevitably he or she would want to either conceal or remove any slave mark, which was not only a reminder to the individual of their past and lowly position in society but also an obvious sign to others of a previous lack of importance in society.

The less drastic option was to conceal the mark under a patch called an *aluta* or *splenium*. These were made of leather softened with alum and came in a variety of shapes, including crescent moons and stars. According to Petronius (AD 27–66), the writer of an early satirical novel, one former slave attempted to conceal a branding on his forehead simply by growing his hair. The more risky option was to have the marks removed. The earliest description of tattoo removal comes from a medical text thought to have been written at the beginning of the sixth century AD by a doctor named Aetios. He suggests applying one of two different mixtures; one of lime or gypsum mixed with sodium carbonate, and the other made from pepper rue and honey. He goes on to describe the method of application and treatment:

> When applying, first clean the tattoo with nitre, smear them with resin of terebinth, and bandage for five days. On the sixth prick the tattoos with a pin, sponge away the blood, and then spread a little salt on the pricks … apply the aforesaid prescription and cover it with a linen bandage. Leave it on five days and on the sixth smear on some of prescription with a feather. The tattoos are removed in twenty days, without great ulceration and without a scar.

This is a process still practised and known nowadays as salubrasion. Contrary to all this, it seems that the early Christian pilgrims wore tattoos as a record of the particular pilgrimage they had undertaken.

The Early Church and Cosmetics

The early Church fathers consistently condemned cosmetics. According to St Clement who lived in the first century AD, 'Thrice I say not once do they deserve to perish who use crocodile excrement and anoint themselves with the froth of putrid humours and stain their eyebrows with soot but their cheeks with white lead'. St Gregory of Nazianus, a fourth century cleric, condemned any use of make-up commending his sister Gorgonia as she 'neither cared to curl her own hair nor to repair her lack of beauty by the aid of a wig'.

However, some churchmen who vigorously expressed their views on make-up, Tertullian (AD 160–AD 220), for example, were not part of the mainstream early Christian Church. Tertullian, in fact, belonged to small sect known as the Montanists. This group was regarded as somewhat heretical and therefore even within the Church itself Tertullian's views would probably have received little attention. While we should not exaggerate the importance of the views expressed by the early churchmen we should not dismiss their statements as worthless either. Look at Clement's condemnation in the example above. While he condemns the wearing of make-up, he does give us some information about what make-up was worn; in this instance, he mentions crocodile dung (which is white), white lead and soot. Also, we can deduce that the early fathers' repeated condemnation of make-up came about because cosmetics were such a common feature of everyday life. This does not, however, detract from the importance of the Church's attitude that opposed make-up in a very vigorous way and which would come to be of considerable influence during the Middle Ages.

Miscellaneous Recipes

Cleopatra's treatment (reputedly) for hair loss:

One part of burnt domestic mice, one part of burnt remnants of vine, one part of burnt horse teeth, one part of bear fat, one part of deer marrow, one part of reed bark. Pound them dry, then add a sufficient amount of honey until the thickness of the honey is convenient, and then dissolve the fat and the marrow, knead and mix them. Place the remedy in a copper box. Rub the alopecia until new hair grows back. Similarly, falling hair should be anointed everyday.

Metradora's face cream:

To make the face bright: Berenice the queen of Egypt, nicknamed Cleopatra, used this. Having thrown the horn of a deer in a new vase, she roasted it in oven and, having removed it, she found it whitened; she crushed it with milk and anointed herself.

Sadly, we know nothing about Metradora, who may not have even been a real person.

Pliny the Elder's recipe for hair remover:

The drops of the vine which are a kind of gum ... act as a depilatory if the hair be repeatedly smeared with them and oil.

3

THE MIDDLE AGES:
EAST MEETS WEST, LITERATURE FOR WOMEN AND THE CHURCH AGAINST COSMETICS

After beautifying the hair, the face ought to be adorned [because] if its adornment is done beautifully it embellishes even ugly women.

The Trotula

Introduction

The term Middle Ages is modern parlance. Broadly speaking, this refers to the period that begins with the Sack of Rome in AD 410 by the Visigoths (an event that signalled the collapse of Roman Empire in the West) and ends with the fall of Constantinople in the East to the Ottoman Turks in AD 1453. Being a span of many hundreds of years, this period is often broken down into the Early Middle Ages, lasting from the fifth to the eleventh centuries, with the term High Middle Ages denoting the twelfth and thirteenth centuries, while the fourteenth and fifteenth centuries are often referred to as the Late Middle Ages. Medieval society was a feudal, male-orientated regime based around noblemen, churchmen and serfs. In the Early Middle Ages people lived in small communities, built around the church and the manor house. In the later medieval period, small towns had begun to emerge, marking a move away from rural communities to living in a more urban setting.

In medieval society, as had been the case in the ancient world, a person's outward appearance was interpreted as a reliable gauge of their social status. One's appearance was also an indication of the moral code one lived by. It is, I think, fair to say that while we recognise that clothing could be an important means of expressing status and even moral standards, the nature and condition of the skin and hair went further, defining an individual's social position and temperament but also offering important clues to his or her physical wellbeing, something not so easily interpreted from what someone might be wearing. This makes the skin and hair as well as the make-up used to protect, to embellish and potentially improve these bodily features, particularly significant.

In the Middle Ages the same materials were used to paint the faces on a painted panel as were used in reality on women's faces. Sometimes the artist who painted the canvas was also the one to paint the actual canvas; that is, the human face. The Italian painter Cennino Cennini (*c* 1370–*c* 1440) reminds his apprentices of this fact: 'In the exercising of your profession you will sometimes have to stain or paint on flesh chiefly to paint the face of a man or a woman'. One twelfth century monk known as the Monk of Montaudon, referring to church figurines and their decoration, even complained that there was 'not enough make-up for these statues because of all the ladies who use rouge'. The same mixtures were being used to paint the blush on art works as were used on women's faces. A poem written in Dutch by Jan Van Boendale in about 1330, or perhaps a few years later, compares works of art to the practice of women painting themselves with cosmetics describing the latter as a bad habit, 'they [the women that is] grease and anoint their faces to appear beautiful and admired by many; but as a painter varnishes an image with all its deceiving decoration shining beautifully as if it were solid gold it is on the inside still wood so a woman has varnished her skin to make it look beautiful and shining it is however still a futile thing, what there is stays the same. That can never change'. The poet may well be referring in particular to the egg-based paint, which was commonly used on painted panels and with which women were known to make up their faces.

There is plenty written about cosmetics at this time, which in itself reflects their continuing and integral existence in everyday life. However, with the pervasive influence of the Christian religion, the burial of artefacts with the deceased no longer occurs, creating a dearth of physical remains; that is, cosmetic implements, containers or their residue. As ever, art work can be ambiguous and any evidence of cosmetics difficult to detect. Therefore, to learn about cosmetics in the medieval period we have to heavily rely on the written record.

Medieval Beauty: The Gold Standard

Much of what is written about beauty in this period is in relation to women. The ideally beautiful medieval woman possessed a high forehead, pale unblemished skin, rosy cheeks, red or pink lips, and a complexion completely free from wrinkles. In the words of one thirteenth century French poet and troubadour, Robert de Blois, who was writing around the middle of the thirteenth century,

> In all women the beautiful face is the most pleasing. A woman who does not have a beautiful face will never be beautiful. A yellow, wrinkled up, and dry face should often be veiled. A beautiful mouth, beautiful teeth, beautiful nose, beautiful eyes, clear complexion should never be veiled.

Although this statement dates from the latter end of the Middle Ages, these features were the essential element of beauty and held good from beginning to the end of the medieval period – and, indeed, beyond. In order to achieve this high standard the practice of applying make-up is thought to have been quite widespread, at least among ladies of the higher social classes, despite the fact that this drew much criticism especially from the Church. Vicente Ferrer (1350–1419) a Dominican friar beatified by the Catholic Church, wrote: 'Is there a lady amongst us who does not wear cosmetics or cream on her face, or uses depilatories ...? How they sorrowfully take off that cream and put on snake and lizard water. Oh, they sin greatly those who act so vainly in order to please men.' The answer, in respect of wealthier women in society, was that probably there was not.

While the perfect facial features admired in the medieval world were much in the classical tradition, ideas about how a woman should wear her hair had changed. Greek and Roman women were required to wear their hair carefully styled. Long loose locks were only appropriate for very young girls, the uncivilised, or those in the throes of mourning a loved one. In contrast, the ideally beautiful woman in medieval times was perceived as having exceptionally long hair, perhaps plaited but remaining in a style which emphasised the great length of her locks. Think of the long hair of Rapunzel in the fairy tale of that name. The tale is, in fact, a much later story but one modelled on the earlier and common 'maiden in the tower' motif that dates from around the tenth century onwards and plays upon the beauty and eroticism of hair. The high forehead favoured from medieval times was a new feature too.

Scorn, as ever, was poured upon women who took too much time over their appearance. This led to the beautiful woman being presented as idle, someone who did not perform any function other than to be looked at. Attending to one's appearance, according to

Geoffrey de la Tour Landry (1330–1402), a nobleman who wrote his *Book of the Knight in the Tower* as a guide to manners for his daughter, 'could make you late for church!' – at a time when that was a cardinal sin. To some extent, spending time in front of a mirror as opposed to doing other things was a practical necessity if a woman was to maintain appearance to the high standard set by those writing about beauty or who depicted the beautiful woman in art. In the medieval period, just as had been the case in the ancient world, make-up needed to be repaired, it was not waterproof so it might run in the rain, but it might also dry up in the sun or simply wear off over the day. Furthermore, to maintain such a model of attractiveness one would hardly be engaged in hard labour; this would soil the hands and tan the skin, neither of which were considered attractive or sexually appealing.

Medieval Men

There is little to link medieval men with make-up although it is likely that they did use some products, as men had done in Greece and Rome for the purposes of hygiene, if not for the aesthetic and religious reasons that men had used make-up in Ancient Egypt or in prehistoric times. Hygiene was important for the purposes of health and the visual projection of the status of men just as it was for women. A man of any standing should smell pleasant in order to disassociate himself from the poor. Other than products used for hygiene purposes, however, cosmetics for men in the medieval period consisted largely of preparations to disguise the appearance of old age such as dye to conceal grey hair, treatments for baldness or to maintain any facial hair when this was in fashion.

The Written and Oral Tradition

In the medieval world, much of the knowledge about particular beauty products and their uses were passed on by word of mouth. Standards of literacy were relatively low. There were some works written in the local vernacular that may have been understandable to people living in a given area where that particular dialect was spoken. On the other hand, the geographical reach of works written in the accepted, formal and universal language of Latin may have had a broader scope. However, given the small percentage of people who could read, oral knowledge passed down from person to person, household to household, remained paramount. Some texts were even intended to be read aloud so that those who could not read could learn from their contents. The *Chastoiement des Dames* (*The Ladies' Instruction*), a rhyming verse of some 700 lines dating from 1260, is one example of such a text. Clearly, the message of care of the body and standards of beauty, particularly pertaining to the female body, was not restricted to those who could read, or afford a book.

Herbals, Household and Conduct Books

In practical how-to books – broadly, herbals, cookery books or books on general household management – recipes (or receipts as they were known at the time) for beauty products were collected together and appeared alongside instructions on how to make all sorts of other things including food, medicines and even household cleaners. For example, we may find information on how to make a skin cream in a book that also gives instructions on how to bake various kinds of cakes or how to brew ale. Herbals contained information about plants with medicinal properties but also referred to their cosmetic uses. However, while cosmetic recipes are found in earlier herbals they became much more common in later works of this kind.

Information about beauty products are also to be found in conduct books. Largely written by men for women, these books were aimed at instructing women in appropriate behaviour in terms of both their religious observance and domestic life. That is to say, conduct books encouraged piety and devotion to one's husband while endeavouring to teach the skills of good household management. As women were expected to conform to a strict code of moral and social behaviour, conduct books tended to rail against the use of cosmetics as indicative of vanity and sexual promiscuity. In his text, *The Book of the Knight of the Tower*, Geoffrey de la Tour Landry dismisses cosmetics forcefully as evil, recounting the following moral tale of a woman who pays too much attention to her appearance:

> What, will this lady never be done combing herself! Staring at herself in the mirror? It proves however to be a mirror of evil omen and as it pleased God to make an example of her even as she stared into the mirror she perceived the enemy who bared his behind so ugly and horrible that the woman lost her reason as if possessed by the devil.

This is pretty strong stuff and, in the medieval period, when the church and religious belief was a powerful influence, the possibility of such a punishment would have been taken quite literally.

It was common for skin creams and other beauty products to be made at home and household management books contained recipes for these to ensure that women, not perhaps the lady of the house herself but more likely her housekeeper and other female servants, knew how to prepare them. No doubt there would have been a good deal of trial and error in the process of making a cosmetic; these preparations were frequently a lengthy process requiring a good number of ingredients with little or no indication of how much to use of each. In reality, these books with their instructions, were a valuable aid to the women of a household.

Cosmetics and the Church

For the most part, the clergy were unrestrained in their condemnation of make-up and there is no doubt that their opinions became much more influential in the Middle Ages than they had been at the latter end of the classical period when the Christian religion was still in its infancy. According to medieval religious ideology, wearing make-up was not only deceitful and immoral – it was a crime against God. Medieval people believed in divine retribution for their sins. One medieval illuminated manuscript attributed to the twelfth century Dominican friar John of Freiberg (from a copy dating from the first half of the fourteenth century) insists that a woman should even be asked at confession whether she 'has plucked hair from her neck or brows or beard for lasciviousness or to please men ... because this is a mortal sin unless she does so to remedy severe disfigurement or so as not to be looked down on by her husband'.

There were, however, a few important members of the church who did speak out in favour of the use of make-up under certain circumstances. For example, Thomas of Aquinas (1224–1274), a respected Italian friar and philosopher, believed that the application of make-up was permissible in order that a wife might maintain her husband's interest, as long as it was not so much as to attract the attention of other men. He also believed that beauty products could, and should, be applied to conceal the ravages of disease. Some men, it seems, were a little more practical and liberal in their ideas and as a result, appear somewhat more gracious towards women in general.

Suffice to say, standards of beauty (that is, a pale skin, a blemish free complexion, a demure blush, attractive lips and beautiful hair) were fixed and for most, any attempt at such perfection was unachievable without the aid of make-up. Women remained under pressure whichever way they turned, to make the best of their looks by whatever means they could. From a woman's point of view, an attractive appearance remained useful in terms of acquiring a husband. Pale skin was not only to be admired for its great beauty but was also seen as evidence of fertility, youth, wealth and general good health; such a woman was therefore a good match.

Popular Literature

In addition to the more academic medical works, serious religious texts or instruction manuals specifically aimed at women, contemporary works of poetry and prose also mention make-up. Popular literature associates the use of cosmetics with beauty or an aspiration to beauty. However, this often leads to the extolling of the virtues of natural beauty while artificial beauty, achieved through the use of cosmetics, is shunned. The courtly romance, as a genre, was popular in the late medieval period. This describes an imaginary world in which ideas of love and of beauty are central themes. While these texts give us little to go on regarding what sorts of make-up were being used and what these might have been made of, the romances are a good guide to what was considered the ideal of beauty at this time, as well as to the ideas that surrounded the possession and the maintenance of an attractive appearance. The medieval romance idealised women, again setting that very high standard for ordinary mortals to achieve. Just as in the classical tradition, beauty is described in terms of the perfect beauty of nature. The *Roman de la Rose* (1237), an allegory of courtly love, is one important example of this genre. The text is the work of two authors and is incomplete. However a good chunk of the work (some 4,058 lines to be precise) has survived. The protagonist is a young man recounting a dream in which he enters a beautiful garden in search of a particular rose. He meets various characters in the garden but the first person he comes across is Oiseuse, who introduces herself to the young man as follows:

All my companions call me Idleness,
A woman rich and powerful am I.
Especially I'm blessed in one respect, have no care except to tress and comb my hair, amuse myself, and take mine ease.

Her skin is pale, of matchless beauty by contemporary standards. However, though her beauty may be admired the physical description of Oiseuse in the poem unfavourably associates make-up and beauty with idleness and self-obsession.

Elsewhere in popular literature others, such as the poet Geoffrey Chaucer (1343–1400), also waxed lyrical about the beautiful woman. Emily in his *Knight's Tale* is so perfect in appearance that her onlookers wonder 'whether she be a woman or goddess'. She possesses a 'fresh beautee' and a 'fairnesse' that would seem to be beyond the reach of women in reality. The lady is like a flower 'that fairer was to see, than is the lily upon his stalk green'. There is no suggestion that she used make-up to achieve such perfection. In the *Physician's Tale* the central character Virginia is also the very personification of natural beauty. Chaucer follows the well trodden theme of preferring natural beauty to artifice, when the latter is defined as the semblance of beauty acquired through the use of make-up. Going further, Chaucer uses cosmetics in his *Canterbury Tales* as a means of demonstrating the shortcomings of some of his characters, their lifestyles and attitudes. He says: 'Beware of being cuckolded by a woman painting her face whose thoughts are far from her marriage carrying a crystalline mirror'. His remarks about make-up express the conventional view that cosmetics were corrupt and those who use them immoral. However, the reader can also extrapolate some more factual information from the comments he makes. Note the lustful carpenter's wife Alisoun in the *Miller's Tale*, who has plucked and darkened her eyebrows. The ugly Summoner, an ecclesiastical court official in *The Summoner's Tale,* whose appearance is described in detail, is apparently suffering from a bad case of acne. Of interest here is Chaucer's detailed list of cosmetics that, in Chaucer's view, would fail to conceal this affliction: 'No quicksilver, lead ointments, tartar creams, no boragic, nor brimstone, so it seems, could make a salve that had the powder to bite, Clean up or cure his whelks [pimples] of knobbly white'.

The Summoner's ugly body is, in fact, the product of his equally unpleasant soul. Although there is no suggestion that the character himself uses make-up, by the inclusion of this list of beauty products Chaucer has left us a few clues as to what women who applied cosmetics might choose to use. Quicksilver (mercury) and lead ointments, both known and used in the Classical period as skin care products, were corrosive and poisonous but despite this continued to be used in the Middle Ages. The other cosmetics in Chaucer's list are much more likely to have some benefit. Nowadays, the herb borage is known to soothe the skin while both brimstone (the archaic name for sulphur) and tartar, an effervescent acid, a by-product of the wine industry, are believed to be effective skin care treatments – still used today.

Art and Artefact

After conversion to Christianity, people were no longer buried with everyday belongings, possessions of value or items of personal significance. As a result, fewer artefacts relating to grooming and the toilette survive from this period, though there are, however, some relevant examples that I can draw to the readers' attention here. The material evidence that survives does so mainly in the form of treasured items that were buried for safekeeping at times of crisis, such as the immediate aftermath of the fall of Rome or the subsequent Viking invasions in the ninth and tenth centuries. These hoards, as they are known, sometimes include items such as mirrors and cosmetic containers made of valuable metals of either silver or gold. The superior quality of these objects is an indication not only of the value of their contents but also suggests cosmetic containers themselves remained highly valued, the visible and tangible trappings of great wealth. The Traprain Law treasure, discovered in East Lothian in Scotland, is a silver hoard from the fifth century AD, probably buried very shortly after the departure of the Romans from Britain. Among the finds at Traprain, there is a vessel which is believed to be a toilette box or container. Although now in poor condition because the piece along with the rest of the hoard has been chopped up perhaps with a view to melting the vessels down, this is an item that would have belonged to a wealthy person belonging to the social elite. A hoard of coins, jewellery and toilette artefacts known as the Erfurt treasure was found in 1998 tucked into a wall cavity in a medieval house in Erfurt in Germany. These valuable possessions were probably stowed there in a hurry by their Jewish owners around the time of the Black Death (1348–1350). Some blamed the Jews for the spread of this disease and so this group were persecuted at this time. Among the items in this hoard there is a silver gilt cosmetic set consisting of a chain with a bottle and accessories attached. The ornate bottle, with its elaborate flower petal stopper, was found to contain cotton fibres soaked with a liquid, which may have been perfume. Of the three small tools attached to the chain, only one, an ear cleaner, has survived without damage. The chain appears to be a rare example of a medieval chatelaine, a set of short chains attached to a woman's belt with useful objects attached. On occasion, keys might be suspended in this fashion, but instruments used for cosmetic purposes were also carried around in this way. However, examples of cosmetic utensils or containers dating from the Middle Ages, whether lavish like these items or simple, remain rare.

Glass mirrors are a common feature in medieval literature even if we don't find too many actual examples. They were usually circular and convex, rather like a large glass bubble. Some had a handle while others were small, indeed similar in size and shape to modern compacts, making them very portable and therefore easy to use anywhere. Glass mirrors were manufactured in Germany, and later, more specifically in the city of Venice. Aside from their use as a looking glass or *speculum*, these were also powerful symbols of magic, good and bad. In a religious context, mirrors were believed to have the power to absorb the goodness from the church and its saints and transfer this to the person in possession of the mirror. Small mirrors, either circular or oval, could be bought at churches for this purpose. However mirrors could also expose flaws. In essence narcissistic, they were believed capable of exposing evil and maintained a mystique that associated them with black magic and the devil. In addition, convex mirrors were used for the more practical purpose of not only viewing one's own reflection but also to project light in order to see one's surroundings. By the later medieval period, mirrors were in widespread use. Some sort of mirror was a common, perhaps even essential, personal possession with the kind of variety of uses such as those I have mentioned. In 1384 records show that more than a thousand mirrors were landed in London by ship, a staggeringly large number and again an indication that these were in common usage. Like mirrors, combs were considered both practical and decorative and even symbolic objects. These were important not only for grooming one's hair but also as a tool for controlling head lice and other infestations. France was an important manufacturer, exporting combs made from ivory or boxwood. The fine craftsmanship on these objects is an indication that these were highly prized possessions.

Although mirrors could be compact and therefore portable and while basic cosmetic tools such as tweezers might be attached to one's belt and combs were small enough to fit in a pocket, it remained unacceptable to repair one's appearance in public. The old woman in the *Roman de la Rose* makes this point clear:

If her complexion loses colour and the heart is tormented as a result she should arrange always to have aqueous ointments hidden in boxes in her chamber for the purposes of painting her face but she must take care that none of her guests can smell or see them.

This would have been considered sound advice in the real world at this time. Just as had been the case in Ovid's day, make-up was intended to be applied behind closed doors. Cosmetics were omnipresent but remained hidden, largely the prerogative of women.

Make-up and Medicine

After the fall of the Roman Empire in the West, the body of medical knowledge that was passed down from antiquity was preserved by those living and working in the eastern half of the old Roman Empire, which became known as the Byzantine Empire. New medical texts began to appear written, this time, in Arabic. Following on from the close relationship that had existed between cosmetics and medicine in the ancient world, beauty products became firmly embedded as a branch of medicine in the Arabic tradition. It was deemed entirely appropriate for the authors of medical texts writing in the medieval period to include creams and ointments and, where appropriate, to stress both the curative qualities of these products and their ability to make someone, more often than not a woman, appear more attractive.

Recipes for skin-care products, hair restorers, hair dyes and various means of hair removal were frequently included in medical manuals. There were even unguents intended to repair the self-mutilation sustained by grieving women like Princess Sichelgaita, a Lombard princess living in the tenth century who is described by the contemporary chronicler William of Apulia as 'ripping her cheeks with her nails and tearing at her dishevelled hair' in distressed frenzy upon the impending death of her husband. It is also true that if one survived a particular disease, the process of the illness itself often left its mark on the skin or the hair. The application of cosmetics had the potential to remedy these flaws. Byzantine medical texts not only preserved the earlier expertise of the Ancient Greek physicians but endeavoured to build upon this knowledge too. A vast output of at least 100 volumes is attributed to one Avicenna (980–1037) also known as Al-Kindi. An Arab physician of Persian origin, Avicenna's *Canon of Medicine*, would remain fundamental to European medical knowledge for a further 700 years after it was originally written. In the second volume of this work, Avicenna lists some simple cosmetics, which had, in addition, he believed, medical uses. He promoted bathing and massage with aromatic ointments and composed one volume entirely on the topic of roses and their precious properties; in fact, his are the first recorded instructions for distilling rosewater. According to Avicenna: 'Bitter almond is used on freckles red spots and other ugly marks on the body'. He noted the benefits of iris and lemon juice for improving the complexion and recommends alum for underarm perspiration. He prescribed arsenic for removing unwanted hair though he also, rather strangely given its use as a depilatory, suggests that arsenic be mixed with pine resin as a cure for baldness. Avicenna includes quite a number of dyes for darkening the hair including bitumen, blackberries or bramble leaves boiled down, mulberry, columbine and even copper. He recommends the use of leaves and berries of the sumac, (a flowering shrub used as a dying agent in the tanning industry), to darken hair, to conceal grey and preserve the appearance of youth. In the Late Middle Ages, medical men moved away from some of Avicenna's ideas. For example, bathing was discouraged in the belief that it opened the pores and let disease in. This resulted in a decline in standards of personal hygiene and, inevitably, an increase in the spread of illness and disease, the very opposite of the intention of a curb on bathing. Albucasis, (936–1013), an eminent Muslim physician and surgeon working in Spain, composed a thirty-volume treatise on medicine. His eleventh book was devoted to cosmetic surgery, including breast reduction, 'nose jobs' and eyelid surgery, while volumes nineteen to twenty five are about cosmetics in general. According to Albucasis, make-up was 'used by women and many men'.

The *Trotula*

The text known to historians as the *Trotula* is an important work on women's medicine. Written around the eleventh or twelfth century, the so-called *Trotula* is in fact not one book, but a collection of three volumes. The work originated from Salerno in southern Italy, a place that, throughout the Middle Ages, was a centre of medical excellence with a world-famous physic garden called The Garden of Minerva, where many plants were grown for their therapeutic benefits and cosmetic use. The third volume of the *Trotula* is often referred to as the *Trotula Minor* or the *Ornatus Mulierum*. It is this volume that takes as its main topic the subject of women's cosmetics. Although the entire three volumes were initially believed to be the work of one woman, recent research has concluded that while one of the books may have been written by an unknown female author, the other two (of which the *Trotula Minor is* one) were probably composed by a man or indeed more than one man. The text, written in Latin, circulated widely from the twelfth to the fifteenth century. It was then translated into the vernacular, presumably testament to the desire for such knowledge. The *Trotula Minor* covers make-up and body care, in head to toe order, very much in the tradition of the Greek doctors from the classical period who used the same format, that is to say, the author deals with hair care, then face, lips, teeth, personal hygiene and so on, describing a mixture of local and imported ingredients and products made from plants and mineral deposits, as well as some animal secretions. The cosmetic treatments specified in this text were often intended to remedy the effects of disease or infection; skin problems and hair loss from disease translate easily to skin care, hair dyes and hair thickeners. Unlike other contemporary works on this subject, such as the early Western medical texts known as leech books, (leech being an early word for physician) or early herbals, which demonstrate a reliance on superstition, incantations and prayers that devalue, for the purposes of this book anyway, some of the material they contain, the contents of the *Trotula Minor* (as with the other two volumes) indicates an extensive practical medical knowledge. The often-complicated preparation of these cosmetics is described in some detail, though only a few of the recipes give specific weights and measures. Also, the *Trotula Minor* even harks back to the comments made by William of Apulia about the Princess Sichelgaita noted above and deals with the subject of self harm, citing a recipe for an unguent that is useful for, among other things, the blemishes on the face which Salernitan women make while mourning the dead. Examples of recipes taken from this work are cited throughout this chapter.

The Flos del Tresor de Beautat

Another medieval manuscript known as *Flos del Tresor de Beautat* (*Flower of the Treasure of Beauty*) is similarly devoted to women's cosmetics and health. This is a late medieval Spanish text written in Catalan. The *Tresor* may have been intended for women of some social standing and as an attempt to offset much misogynistic literature in vogue at the time. However, unlike the *Trotula Minor*, the text and the knowledge it contained probably attracted a limited audience. Given the language in which it was written, its instruction would have little circulation beyond Northern Spain. This is really a local self-help book that preserves in its pages recipes for perfumed products, skin peelers, whiteners, hand creams and hair dyes. The text is unusual in that many of the recipes it contains use animal body parts or secretions. Herbs and flowering plants are the more common ingredients in make-up at this time, with few exceptions. However, while dog's faeces used in face creams, for example, or pigs' nails ground to a powder and used as a teeth whitener seem distasteful to us, these were at least relatively easy to obtain. Indeed, of the animal products used in make-up in the *Tresor*, the anal gland secretion, civet, added to cosmetics as a fixative, and the grease from sheep's wool (lanolin), are still used in modern cosmetics.

Medieval Trade

Constantinople, Baghdad, Venice and other towns in Northern Italy, Cordoba in southern Spain, and the French ports of Dieppe and Calais were all great trading centres in the Middle Ages. Goods used as cosmetics or ingredients in cosmetics came via these centres as part of the market in luxury items. Expensive aromatic products were imported from Asia and Africa at some cost for use as cosmetics as well as having a medicinal function. Certain trading centres became known as the best place to source particular types of make-up of quality. For example, apricot face cream was distributed via Dieppe and Calais, and red lead for use as rouge at markets in southern Spain. Flower water from Byzantium and Baghdad and other scented products were brought to the West by those returning from the Crusades. Following the Crusades, rose water in particular became increasingly popular for bathing as well as for washing hands; the better-off in medieval society adopted a fashion, brought back from the East by the crusaders, for providing rose water for visitors, who were encouraged to wash their hands at the table before eating and also in between courses. Roses were believed to originate in Ancient Persia and were highly valued in the medieval period for their scent and their exotic history, and were understood to have both medicinal and hygiene benefits, as well as being a popular if rather luxurious ingredient in beauty products. In fact, there had been a flourishing industry in cultivated roses for use in perfumes and cosmetics as well as garlands for the hair in Italy since at least Roman times. The crusaders also introduced Eau de Chypre, toilette water that included rose water mixed with stryrax, a gum resin and certain herbs. This originated in Cyprus, an island captured during the Crusades by Richard the

Lionheart. Merchants and itinerant pedlars sold these goods across the western world. An extant thirteenth century French poem describes a pedlar selling a variety of goods to improve a lady's appearance including, 'razors, tweezers, looking glasses, toothbrushes, toothpicks, bandeaus and curling irons, ribbons, combs, mirrors, rosewater ... cotton with which they rouge themselves and whitening with which they whiten themselves'. There isn't much detail here as to what was being used to whiten the skin or as far as the ingredients of the rouge are concerned. Nevertheless, these few short lines do give us an insight into the sort of goods available even from itinerant sellers. Buying from pedlars and travelling merchants at fairs or door-to-door would indicate a rather sporadic supply for these goods but these small-time merchants must have found a market that made selling them of financial benefit.

In the fourteenth and fifteenth centuries more manufactured or finished goods were being traded in Europe. In the main, however, beauty products continued to be assembled in the home, especially the homes of the wealthy. Home-produced make-up might be a cheaper option, especially if the ingredients were home-grown or if the cosmetic was made from foodstuffs that the household already grew or perhaps bought in for cooking. Indeed, the by-products of food preparation were sometimes recycled for use, for example, as a skin cream; a recipe for skin care product might include chicken fat or perhaps ox bile. Other readily available materials that could be gathered rather than purchased could also form the basis of an accepted beauty treatment. Crow's eggs, beaten to a pulp, were applied to dye the hair black. Not only the faeces of dogs, already noted, but also of rats were considered effective treatments for hair loss. It seems that even for those women and men who were relatively poor, there were cosmetic products and the knowledge as to how to use them available – should they have the opportunity and the wish to do so.

The Black Death

In the medieval period serious illness was a common occurrence and a constant concern. Where a disease was not fatal, the physical evidence of having suffered from it, such as scars, pockmarks and hair loss needed to be covered up with make-up so that the vision of a now-healthy individual could be presented to the world. During the scourge of the Black Death, the plague that swept through Europe in the thirteenth century, perfumed waters, pomanders and other scented ointments became very popular. Pleasant smells allowed individuals to cope with the stench of death; amber apples made from musk, a black powdery sap called aloe, (the plant genus to which aloe vera belongs), camphor (a waxy, solid and strong-smelling tree resin) and rosewater were worn around the neck. Doctors wedged a pomander into the top of their cane when visiting patients; hence the shape of the doctor's cane in later history. Not only did the pleasant smell help to mask the disagreeable odour of ill health, those living at this time also believed that pleasant smells might counteract the spread of the disease itself. Plagues such as the Black Death were believed to be transmitted by bad air. This was based on an earlier Greek medical theory and known as miasma, the Greek word meaning pollution. Undoubtedly aromatic herbs and pomanders would have helped to counteract the smell of death and decay that surrounded the living but we no longer place any store on the potential of fragrances to provide protection against bacterial or viral disease, even when that bacterial or viral infection is carried in the air.

Make-up and Hygiene

Health and hygiene were especially important in an age when many diseases could be fatal. Bathing to keep clean and ward off disease was recommended in the medical texts books of the Arabic doctors. The author of the *Trotula Minor* too favoured bathing. In fact. in the early and middle medieval periods people bathed more than they would do in later centuries. Given some of the mixtures that people were applying directly to their bodies (those dogs' or rats' faeces, for example), taking a bath would have been most advisable. Avicenna devoted a whole chapter to smelling pleasant, something which bathing and the use of herbs could achieve. The aromatic oils he promoted are still popular today; herbs such as coriander, for example, are now known to have some antibacterial value. Soap was used for washing clothes but toilet waters (made from myrrh, roses or perhaps orange blossom) were used to cleanse the body. Because, in the latter years of the Middle Ages many began to believe that bathing was a dangerous fad and that a cold bath could be the death of you before you even reached home, people, particularly the wealthier in society (who could afford these things), used flower waters to keep themselves clean. These waters were also intended to mask any body odour that resulted from lack of personal hygiene and the infrequency with which people changed their clothes or indeed took a bath. Other toilet waters in use included the so-called Queen of Hungary's water (which originally dates from around 1370) and was applied as a sort of cure-all; that is to say, one could take a bath in it but there was also a belief that water could also be drunk, inhaled or rubbed on the surface of the skin Whether it was consumed or applied, Hungary Water was believed to be not only effective against disease but also to preserve youth. The earliest recipes for this water include alcohol (perhaps brandy) and rosemary to refresh the skin. Its name is a bit of a mystery, though legend has it that it was created for the aging Queen of Hungary to restore her youthful looks. Having applied it, despite being seventy years old, the queen received a marriage proposal – apparently such was its effectiveness. Sweet powders were also very popular for keeping the body smelling pleasant. These came at a price. There is record of Margaret, Duchess of Clarence, or perhaps her husband, purchasing a selection of sweet powders including the popular citronade, a mixture of sugar and citrus used as a face whitener and a pomade (a waxy substance used to style one's hair) at the price of 37s 8d, a princely sum at the time.

Skin Care

Taking care of one's skin was important to both sexes but women, in particular, strived for an unsullied pale face and delicate white hands. Much of the body was covered, making the latter particularly important. Those with pure white unblemished hands showed no signs of manual labour so were the moneyed classes. Hands were exposed both to view and to the harsh elements of wind and rain. Something had to be done to preserve their appearance. The *Trotula Minor* recommends, 'for whitening and smoothing the hands let some ransoms (wild garlic) be cooked in water until all the water has been consumed and stirring well add tartar and afterward two eggs and with this you will rub the hands'.

Apart from her hands, a beautiful woman was often described as generally 'faire' meaning not only pale skinned but possessing a clear complexion free from any blemish. Every effort was made to rid the complexion of, or conceal, marks or blemishes, not only marks left by disease, infection or lack of hygiene but also defects such as birthmarks, wrinkles or other signs of aging, moles and even freckles. It was important to remove these blemishes not only to look young, to draw attention to one's social status and good moral character, but to keep in line with contemporary religious ideas – skin blemishes were thought to be the mark of the devil.

As youth was a prerequisite of beauty, anti-aging creams were much in demand at this time, just as they are today. Eglantine rose, also known as sweet briar (a wild rose), and the herb mallow were applied to combat dry skin. The roots of lily, in itself a symbol of great beauty in biblical parable and as a chivalric emblem, were ground up and used as an anti-aging treatment. Women laid soft leather strips soaked with oil and wax on their foreheads overnight to guard against wrinkles. Strawberry or cucumber juice could be applied to clear the complexion. The rather more expensive, indeed exclusive, option of rubbing an amethyst dampened with saliva (one's own presumably) on any offending spots and blemishes was an option for those who had money to spend.

In the Arabic medical tradition, recipes for cleansing (sometimes with the dual purpose of whitening the face) include one that is a mix of flours made from lupins, broad beans and lentils. Another recipe consists of barley bran, watermelon seeds, broad beans, chickpeas and gum resin. Both of these mixtures would have been useful in exfoliating, that is removing dirt and dead skin, from the body's surface even if these would not have been very effective in the removal of any more permanent blemishes such as freckles or birthmarks. The *Trotula Minor* records a face cream made from barley. Again, the coarse grains would have had an astringent effect, removing any dead or loose skin. The herb bisort, an ingredient in some medieval skin treatments, would have had a similar effect. Some face packs were made from exotic and expensive aromatic resin such as frankincense, a resin understood, then and now, as being excellent in combating dry skin and restoring its moisture. As I have already mentioned, frankincense was highly valued by the Ancient Egyptians and a well-established anti-aging treatment in the classical world. Alternatively, a face pack made from the rather-less-appealing and less-fragrant bird dung was an option for the poorer in society. According to Banks' popular herbal, 'Rosemary leaves boiled in white wine made a lady faire of face'. Aloe was used as a moisturiser. The mallow herb was believed to be an effective treatment for dry skin. The following wax substance is prescribed for daily use by the writer of the *Trotula Minor*;

Let oil of violets or rose oil with hen's grease be placed in a clay vessel so that it boils, let very white wax be dissolved then let egg white be added and let powder of well powdered and sifted white lead be mixed in, and again be cooked a little. Then let it be strained through a cloth and to this strained cold mixture let camphor nutmeg and three or four cloves be added. Wrap the whole thing in parchment.

There is a further instruction to keep this mixture until it smells good. The process of making this is certainly time-consuming. There is no indication as to how much was made at one time. Many of its ingredients have a very strong smell and another, that is the lead, is nothing other than dangerous. Daily use of this mixture is unlikely to have had any positive effect in the long term.

Foundation

Women whose skin appeared dark or swarthy would be immediately judged as belonging to the lower ranks of society. For the upper classes being 'fair of face' with not only a pale skin tone but also clear skin was nothing short of essential. A ground wheat powder could be applied to lighten skin tone. Wheat powder was sometimes mixed with pulverised garden lovage, an aromatic herb widely grown as food flavouring and therefore readily available from the kitchen garden. Sour milk was used to whiten not only one's complexion but as a lotion to improve the skin colour over the whole of one's body. According to the *Trotula Minor*,

There is a white make-up that is very easy to make. Put pure wheat in water for fifteen days, then grind and blend it in the water. Strain through a cloth and let it crystallise and evaporate you will obtain a make-up which will be as white as snow. When you want to use it mix it with rose water and spread it on your face which has first been washed with warm water. Then dry your face with a cloth.

Even if this mixture was easy to make, the length of the process was quite extensive. Again, no quantities are given. The phrase 'when you want to use it' suggests that this cosmetic could be stored for some time. Therefore, perhaps making a large amount at once was one practical option. Pulverised ginger was another substance that could not only remove blemishes but also lighten one's skin tone. In fact, this is still used in cosmetic products today to lighten the skin. The *Trotula Minor* recommends applying crushed roots of lily mixed with egg whites and then rinsing the mixture off. Just as interesting as the composition of this cosmetic is the fact that the text implies that roots of lily should be taken by the women to the baths and there mixed with the egg whites, washing the mixture off on leaving; an example of a home-made product used in a public place.

Fashionable women favoured an attractive sheen to the skin. At the very beginning of the medieval period, there were products such as the 'soap' used by the Patrician Pelagia, that promised this effect. The recipe for this is preserved in the writings of Aetius of Amida, a sixth century author.

Soap the Patrician [that is, noble] Pelagia used to make her face shine: Gallic soap, 6 ounces; starch, 1½ ounce; white lead, 1½ ounce; mastic, ½ ounce; deer marrow, 1 ounce; white native sodium carbonate, 4 pastilles; white wax, 3 ounces. Soak the soap beforehand in water in a small jar for five days, changing the rain water every day and filtering the soap. After that, on the sixth day, put the soap in a new cooking pot with the rain water; place on coals, on a low heat, until the soap has melted. Then sprinkle with the wax and the marrow, and when they are dissolved, take the frying pan and stir well with a spittle and sprinkle the mastic and the starch, ground beforehand. Then add the white lead (ground beforehand in some water) in a small dish and beat up with the hand vigorously. Then place in a new jar and use generously.

Unusually, this recipe gives measures and takes the name of a woman who was once a prostitute but who was subsequently made a saint by the Catholic Church, strangely linking the saucy and the sanctified together, if indeed that is the reference that is being made here. An egg-based make-up used in the Middle Ages created a glazed lustrous look and perhaps suggested the glow of divinity possessed by the gods and goddesses of the ancient world, a perfection that was still highly sought-after in the Middle Ages. From the fourteenth century, that is at the later end of the medieval period, crushed mother of pearl, an iridescent powder made form the crushed inner shell of molluscs, had become popular as a face powder. However, the added sparkle that resulted from the application of mother of pearl did not come cheap; this was an option for wealthy women only.

The exactness of the written and physical description of true beauty for women remained as elusive as ever and the toxic nature of at least some of the ingredients in medieval face creams and powder would certainly have done more harm than good. The merits of others simply remain a mystery or even, as in the case of the following recipe, seem counterproductive to the contemporary concept of beauty. The ninth century *Leech Book of the Bald* states: 'That all the body may be of clean and glad and bright hue take oil and dregs of old wine equally much and put them into a mortar and mingle well together and smear the body with this in the sun'. Surely the oil in this would have attracted the sun's rays and tanned the skin. The explanation is probably that this method of caring for one's skin was intended for men and not women.

Rouge

For a woman just a hint of rosy pink on the cheeks was not only considered as attractive as ever but implied health, potential fertility and good morals. Even the precise shade was important. The English physician Gilbertus Angelicus (1180–*c* 1250) in his seven-volume *Compendium of Medicinme,* written around 1240, recommends brazilwood chips with rosewater to redden a lady's cheeks. Brazilwood, or redwood, is used today in brown hair dyes and produced a red-brown shade when used in medieval times as rouge. Gilbertus also recommended that if a lady's cheeks were too red, she could soften the colour by applying the roots of the pleasantly scented cyclamen flower. The ground leaves of the herb angelica, the crushed dried red and orange flowers of safflower and crushed berries of various sorts were also worn as rouge. Cochineal, a bright red dye extracted from crushed insects, was not only useful as rouge but was also thought to possess healing properties. The *Trotula Minor* goes into more detail of how rouge was actually made: 'Here a mixture of brazilwood, alum, egg white and rose water might be applied let her anoint some cotton and press it on her face and it should make her red'. The method of application and even the ingredients seem almost modern.

Hair

Hair could be plucked, dyed, lost and augmented. Of all her natural features, a woman's hair was considered especially erotic and therefore a dangerous temptation to men. For this reason, well-born women covered their hair in public and to expose one's hair suggested a lowly social status or even employment in the sex trade. In art and literature where the suggestion of eroticism might well be intended, women often appeared with their hair in long plaits sometimes with the addition of hair pieces made from flax, wool, cotton or even silk. There were also recipes to thicken or lengthen one's own natural hair. Facial hair was also a means of defining the male gender. Men could purchase expensive perfume that allegedly caused beards to grow.

The *Trotula Minor* recommends that: 'In order to have thick hair, cook willow leaves then grind them blend with olive oil and spread on your hair.' In addition, to encourage one's own hair to grow long, the *Trotula Minor* gives us the following recipe:

> Grind root of marsh mallow with pork grease and you should make it boil for a long time in wine. Afterwards put in well ground cumin and mastic and well cooked egg yolks and mix them together a little. After they have been cooked strain through a linen cloth and set it aside until it becomes cold. Then take the fatty residue which floats on the top and having washed the head well you should anoint it with it.

After applying what one imagines, in this case, would be a rather sticky and pungent concoction, the lady might well wish to comb her hair with a rather more pleasant mixture of dried roses, clove, nutmeg and galangal (a plant root) mixed with rose water. This powder is also recommended by the writer of the *Trotula* who comments that once this has been sprinkled on a lady's hair and combed through, her locks 'will smell marvellously'.

One Arabic text describes a hair dye that could last up to a year made from antimony, ammoniac (an aromatic gum resin) gum Arabic (otherwise known as acacia gum) and gallnuts (from oak trees). This doesn't seem to take any account of the hair growing and the undyed roots showing.

Hair Removal

Medieval art depicts women without any body hair, just as had been the case in the ancient world. This was considered attractive. The removal of hair from the body was also practised, again as it had been in earlier centuries, for reasons of hygiene. Medieval ladies favoured a high hairline too. This fashion is well attested in medieval art as well as in the literature of the period. Vinegar and quicklime were applied to heighten the hairline, basically eroding it and, again due to the caustic nature of the substances applied, often taking the skin with it. What is not clear is which came first – a fashion for a high hairline or the hair loss caused by some of the dangerous cosmetics applied to the face.

Removing unwanted hair helped prevent unpleasant body odour, infestation and disease. Tweezers and razors, which could be used to remove hair, are often found attached to medieval chatelaines, an indication that these tools were often to hand for regular everyday use. Apart from using these tools, there were various cosmetic concoctions that could be applied for this purpose. Some hair removers contained both arsenic (orpiment) and quicklime. As these are very corrosive substances, their ability to remove body hair is not in doubt. However, such a caustic mixture could remove the surface of the skin as well as the unwanted hair if one was not very careful. The writer of the *Trotula Minor* acknowledges this and includes the following instructions for what to do if this happens:

> If the skin is burnt by this depilatory take populeon (a compound recipe including poplar bud) with rose or violet oil or with juice of house leek and mix them until the heat is sedated then anoint the burned area with *ungentum album* (white ointment largely white lead and oxidised lead [yellow] with added scent) until the heat is sedated.

However, it seems that the treatments for the initial damage done by the hair remover includes the application of one further dangerous product; that is, lead. Cinnamon bark, a much safer and more agreeable alternative, was also used as a hair remover. The rough surface of the bark would have exfoliated the skin removing any hair while giving off a pleasant scent. The *Trotula Minor* even advises the reader that if a woman rubs a mixture of ants' eggs, red orpiment (also known as realgar), an arsenic sulphide mineral and gum of ivy onto her skin this will permanently remove unwanted body hair.

Hair Loss

We come across plenty of methods for reversing hair loss in medieval literature. Barley bread, or an application of laurel or myrtle, were all natural products believed to encourage hair to grow again. In fact, the essential oils from laurel and myrtle are still used today to encourage hair growth and prevent hair loss. In order to improve the general condition as well as the thickness of one's hair, the *Trotula Minor* states 'take equal quantities of olive oil, honey and alum. Blend them and add quicksilver more than each of the other ingredients and spread it on several times'. Should a woman begin to lose her hair the writer of the courtly romance *Roman de la Rose* has some advice: 'if (a lady) sees her beautiful blonde hair is falling out (a most mournful sight) ... she should have the hair of some dead woman brought to her or pads of light coloured silk and stuff it all into false hairpieces.' Much in the tradition of the early Church fathers who expressed their views on such matters (Clement of Alexandria and St Gregory of Nazianus. for example) the medieval church took a dim view of wig wearing. According to Saint Bernard of Clairvaux (1090 –1153), 'The woman who wears a wig commits a mortal sin.' To make one's hair look thicker, it could be curled by using tongs heated over a fire. There were also lotions also for making the hair curly. Again, according to the *Trotula Minor*, 'Grind root of danewort with oil and anoint the leaf and tie it on the head with leaves'. Danewort is another word for the dwarf elder. To our taste, this shrub has an unpleasant smell. It had been common practice to paint or gild mirrors and combs made of boxwood with quicksilver or liquid mercury. Sensibly, however, in 1324 this was forbidden in Paris. As the city was a leader in fashion trends, this no doubt helped to curb this dangerous practice. Mercury would have proved not only detrimental to one's hair but also one's overall health.

Hair Dye

Blonde hair was certainly popular in the Middle Ages just as it had been in ancient Greece and Rome. Chaucer compares the hair of his character Virginia in *The Physician's Tale* with the beauty of nature. Virginia has 'tresses resembling the rays of [Phoebus] burnished sunbeams'. This gives us an idea of just how high the bar was set. Nature was perfection and women, in particular, had to strive to equal its colour and beauty with artifice (that is, cosmetics) that were both effective and unnoticed. There were many different plants from which dye to tint hair blonde could be extracted. These included celandine, agrimony, a flowering yellow herb also known as liverwort, boxwood, burnt grape vine ash and saffron which, throughout history, was an expensive commodity. The sap of the Dragon Tree produced a red-gold colour and apart from hair dye was also used for healing purposes, in the process of mummification, in toothpastes, and woodwork, including violin making. Madder, a red plant dye, also dyed hair strawberry blonde. Many of these dyes involved a lengthy process of preparation. This is certainly the case with the following example, again from the *Trotula Minor*:

> For colouring the hair so that it is golden. Take the exterior shell of a walnut and the bark of the tree itself and cook them in water and with this mix alum and oak apples and with these mixed things you will smear the head.

This was just the start of a long process, which involved bandaging the head for the following two days and then a applying a further colouring lotion made from oriental crocus, dragon's blood (resin from the Dragon Tree) and henna mixed with brazilwood. After another three days, the mixture is washed off to reveal a long-lasting blonde. It would be encouraging to think after all that, that the results were as long lasting as the recipe claims.

Blonde was certainly not the only shade coveted by medieval women. Thick dark hair was also admired. The *Trotula Minor* states that, 'If a woman wishes to have long and black hair takes a green lizard and having removed its head and tail cook it in common oil. Anoint the head with this oil. It makes the hair long and black'. Black Henbane also dyed hair black; the contrast of a lady's dark hair against a flawless pale skin was nothing short of erotic.

Eyes and Eyebrows

Eye make–up was not widely used in the Middle Ages though belladonna (which literally translates as 'beautiful lady'), extracted from the perennial plant known commonly as deadly nightshade, was dropped into the eyes to make the pupils dilate and appear large. Belladonna taken internally is a deadly poison and even simply dropped into the eye has the potential to cause long-term blurred vision. However, it does undoubtedly have the effect of dilating the pupils and is still sometimes used by ophthalmologists for this purpose when carrying out eye examinations. Although eye make-up was not in vogue at this time, some women in the medieval period paid attention to the appearance of their eyes by plucking their eyebrows. In Chaucer's *Canterbury Tales* (*The Miller's Tale* to be precise) the carpenter's wife has plucked and darkened her eyebrows as was the fashion: 'Fine plucked were her two brows and like a bow, bended they were and black as any sloe' However, in the medieval romance *Roman de la Rose*, *Beautee*, the personification in terms of appearance of the perfect woman, has not, unlike the carpenter's wife, plucked her eyebrows.

Lips

For colour the *Trotula Minor* recommends rubbing the lips with the bark of the root of the nut tree. Crushed berries were also used. Red plant material (from roots or berries) was mixed with lanolin to produce a somewhat subtler pink shade of lip colour, intended to suggest the wearer was of a more demure character than a lady who might sport a more obvious bright red. Pink lip colour was also somewhat more sophisticated in its composition, being not merely a simple cosmetic but a compound mixture, and so was favoured by better-class women. In Italy in the thirteenth century, lipstick was a key indication of social status – pink shades for the upper classes and the more basic brown-red for the lower rungs of society. While the colour of one's lips might be important, it was no less crucial for a lady at least to keep her lips moist. Beeswax was applied, as it is nowadays, to this end. Albucasis mentions a lip balm made of 'sweet smelling grease that will keep the lips and hands from chapping and make them moist and soft'. In fact, his lip balm was made of suet, marjoram and wine. As ever, the preparation process was complex and lengthy. The suet and marjoram had to be made into balls, which were then sprinkled with wine and kept for twenty-four hours in an airtight container, then cooked in water and strained. The whole process had to be completed four or five times before finally adding some more suet and a little musk or civet (both strong smelling animal scents) to make the product, more appealing to contemporary tastes.

Toothpowders and Breath Fresheners

White clean teeth were a sign of wealth, while black decayed teeth were an indication of poverty. Halitosis or bad breath inevitably accompanied rotting teeth. In the *Roman de la Rose* one of *Beautee*'s appealing features is her fresh breath, 'Her breath was sweet and pure, bathed with mint and thyme'. These aromatic flavours and smells would have certainly been preferable to the vestiges of stale food and wine. The poet Robert de Blois states that; 'If the woman has bad breath she should refrain from breathing on anyone she was conversing with'. This was no doubt sound practical advice. There were, however, treatments to counteract bad breath too. Eating marrow was believed to be beneficial. In Gilbertus Angelicus' *Medical Compendium*, aids to freshen breath include a pepper and salt tooth scrub and pills made from sweet-smelling spice. The Anglo Saxons used chalk to polish teeth and twigs to clean them. A cosmetic brush was excavated in 1941 by the Oxford University Archaeology Society from Purwell Farm at Cassington, Oxfordshire. All that survives is a bronze tube but this would have held a bundle of hairs, like a brush. Those who could afford it, brushed their teeth with aloe and myrrh - both are anti-bacterial. Hildegard of Bingen (1098–1179), a German abbess, in her work *Physica* mentions brushing with aloe and myrrh. Myrrh, being an analgesic may also have eased the pain of toothache. While pig's nails ground to a powder used as tooth whiteners were cheaper and certainly abrasive, these would have been more likely to harbour bacteria than dispel any infection. Gilbertus Angelicus' advice was that everyone should clean their teeth after every meal. The writer or writers of the *Trotula Minor* advocate cleaning the teeth after a main meal, while the Byzantine physician Ioannes Actuarius (1275–1328) mentions tooth whiteners; in order to keep her teeth white, the woman should wash her mouth after dinner with very good wine. Then, 'she ought to dry [her teeth] very well and wipe [them] with a new white cloth. Finally let her chew each day fennel or lovage or parsley, which is better to chew because it gives off a good smell and cleans good gums and makes the teeth very white'.

The *Trotula Minor* includes the following recipe:

For whitening black teeth and strengthening corroded or rotted gums and for a bad smelling mouth, this works best. Take some each of cinnamon, clove, spikenard, mastic, frankincense, grain, wormwood, crab foot, date pits and olives. Grind all these and reduce them to a powder then rub the affected areas.

Such a mixture may not have done much harm, maybe even a little good given the analgesic qualities of clove. Indeed cinnamon is still used in some toothpaste today. (Note that recipes that called for a considerable variety of ingredients or those of the best quality [very good wine as in this recipe, for example] were, and some still are, expensive; such things were not available to the poor).

And Finally ... the Darker Side of Cosmetics

The deliberate misuse of make-up for sinister purposes was not unknown. For example, there is the case of Amadeus VII, the red Count of Savoy (1360–1391); his physician was accused of poisoning him, on the instructions of his mother, by applying an ointment that claimed to thicken hair. Beggars were accused of using make-up almost as actors might to feign leprosy to beg for money. Certainly, medieval cosmetics could be dangerous. Their composition made them ripe for abuse. In later centuries make-up would be exploited to nefarious ends too, as will be decribed.

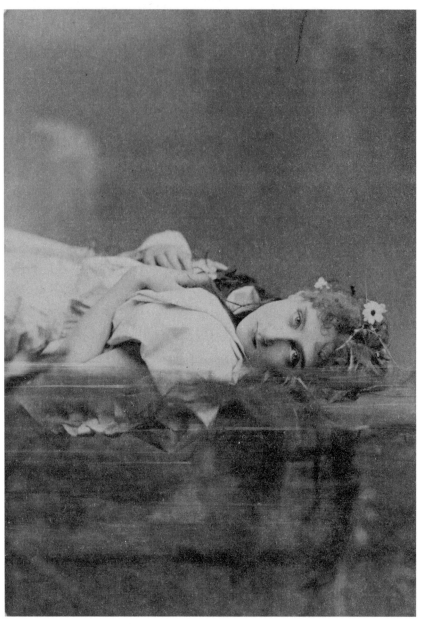

Ophelia on Broadway, *c.* 1890–1910 (Rijksmuseum)

'I have heard of your paintings too, well enough.
God has given you one face and you make yourselves another.
You jig and amble, and you lisp...'

Hamlet, Act 3, Scene 1

4

THE LATE FIFTEENTH AND SIXTEENTH CENTURIES:
THE CLASSICAL REVIVAL, BOOKS OF SECRETS AND THE PRINTING PRESS

On female beauty ...

Cheeks should be fair, have a glow like ivory...the bosom must be white ... forehead spacious (pumiced), wide, high, fair, and serene ... ebony eyebrows of soft short hair ... dark tan or nut brown eyes.

Firenzuola, Dialogue (1548)

And on the appearance of men ...

[Man] must not embellish himself like a woman, for his adornments will then contradict his person as I see some men do, who put curls in their hair and beards with a curling iron and who apply so much make-up to their faces neck and hands that it would be unsuitable for any young wench, even for a harlot who is more anxious to hawk her wares and sell them at a price.

Giovanni Della Casa, Galateo (1558)

Introduction

The period known as the Renaissance traces its origins back to the Italian city of Florence in the fourteenth century, but it was not until the sixteenth century that Europe, as a whole, became enveloped by this movement, which means literally 'rebirth'. The Renaissance, in the eyes of men (and women) of learning, was, first and foremost, a revival of all things classical, particularly in respect of art, literature and philosophy. In addition to this being a period that harked back to the past, however, the Renaissance was also an age of new inventions and discoveries prompted, in part at least, by a growing enthusiasm and respect for trade and commerce. All of this had an effect on the market for make-up, both in terms of what was available and who used it, as well as the extent and even the very nature of the application of the make-up itself. That is to say, cosmetics became very popular, helped by the increasing variety and accessibility of the products on sale. In addition, the invention of the printing press by Johannes Gutenberg around 1440 had begun to make recipes for cosmetics as well as instruction on what sort of make-up to wear, and how to apply these products, more widely available. The use of certain beauty treatments migrated and spread across countries finding their way across Western Europe not only through the increased circulation of written texts but by other means too. Ideas and fashions with regards to appearance spread by word of mouth but also through the movement of people themselves – the mingling of different cultures introduced various ideas about beauty and cosmetics that were influential across Europe. One example of the latter is the story of one Estefania, a woman from Barcelona who moved, with her husband, in 1535 to the court of Empress Isabel of Portugal. She wrote to her mother asking her to send her a jar of *unguentum cetrinum,* a face cream to treat pimples and redness, initially for her own use and that of a friend. In November 1536 Estefania requested further recipes from her mother, which she notes as 'very profitable'. We don't know if this information simply raised her status at court or whether there was any monetary profit being made. She does, however, further request a recipe for cosmetic oil for use by the empress herself.

Make-up was worn largely by women but also by some men at this time. It was elite women, however, especially those who belonged to the English and French courts that set the fashion of the day. The wealthy members of European society generally had the money to buy the more costly products on the market and to follow the latest trends. In fact, the rich continued to wear expensive make-up more as a mark of status than a definition of gender. By the sixteenth century, however, the use of cosmetics had begun to spread beyond the upper classes to the middle rungs of society. These middle classes wanted to show off their new-found affluence, largely acquired through their own successful business enterprises which, in some cases at least, included the direct involvement in the purchase and sale of beauty products or the ingredients to make them. The dilemma that revolved around cosmetics in the late fifteenth and sixteenth centuries was no longer centred on whether or not to wear make-up *per se* but instead focused on the question of what one should wear or perhaps which product or colour one should choose. Such was the enthusiasm for these goods that sumptuary legislation, laws intended to curb excess, had to be passed from time to time to restrict their use.

References to cosmetics in the contemporary literature, whatever the genre, are plentiful but in works of art any evidence for the use of make-up is much less obvious. However, we do know that as men were very often painted sporting beards in sixteenth century portraiture there was a fashion for facial hair. This would have required some maintenance and on occasion, at least, involved some topical treatment that could be called cosmetic. Women, on the other hand, were largely idealised in works of art with a view to adding to a lady's beauty and more specifically concealing any signs of aging. Objects that survive from this period are few but often lavish, reflecting the value, in every sense of the word, placed on make-up and the importance of caring for and maintaining one's appearance.

Physical and Moral Beauty

The ideas surrounding humoral medicine formulated by Galen in the second century AD still held good. According to his terminology, women could be described as cold and wet while men were hot and dry. In Galenical theory the skin was viewed as a protective covering, a link between the exterior and the interior if you like. The Italian poet Firenzuola (1493–1543), in his book *On the Beauty of Women*, first published in 1548, a work which takes the form of a dialogue between a young gentleman and four upper-middle-class women, makes this point by putting the following words into the mouth of Celso, the young gentleman: 'Health produces a bright and lively complexion that outwardly reveals its presence within the body.' There was a fascination with the morality as well as the aesthetic appeal and the physical nature of beauty. The *Book of the Courtier*, an Italian work dating from 1528 and again written in the form of a dialogue, purports to describe the conventions of court life. The author Castiglione, who was not only a writer but also a diplomat and a member of the royal court himself, states that: 'Only rarely does an evil spirit dwell in a beautiful body and so outward beauty is a sign of inner goodness'. In short, while beauty continued to be understood as an expression of one's status, this was also seen as a clearly visible physical metaphor of the health and morality of any given individual, whether male or female.

Feminine Beauty

For women the fashion was for a pale, almost translucent, complexion with shaved eyebrows and a high forehead. Blonde hair or perhaps to be more accurate, strawberry blonde, was popular. A lady's hands and face, in particular, had to look good as they signalled at a glance her status, health and moral wellbeing to the onlooker, especially at a time when heavy clothing concealed much, if not all, of the rest of the body. The beauty of women, where this achieved perfection, was regularly compared with features that belonged to the natural world including lilies, roses and even pearls. Ironically these were also natural ingredients found in contemporary make-up. If women were using cosmetics in this period to best effect, their use should be subtle. Make-up had to be applied skilfully and carefully so that onlookers should wonder at a lady's beauty not knowing whether it was truly natural or enhanced by artificial means, which when obvious, were rather less in favour. The poet John Donne (1572–1631) explains the dilemma with the following comment; 'what thou lovest in her face is colour, and painting gives that, but thou hates it not because it is, but because though knowest it'.

In his *Book of the Courtier* Castiglione remarks: 'Surely you realise how much more graceful a woman is who if indeed she wishes to do so paints herself so sparingly and so little that whoever looks at her is unsure whether she is made-up or not in comparison with one whose face is so encrusted that she seems to be wearing a mask and who dare not laugh for fear of causing it to crack.' Here the writer draws our attention not only to the lack of aesthetic appeal of a woman wearing too much make-up but also to the difficulty of expressing emotion when wearing thick foundation or powder and the disastrous effect on her appearance should she smile or frown. This was certainly one of the more pressing practical problems that arose for a woman who overdid her foundation. Youth continued to be a key factor when looking good. Wrinkles were not simply the superficial signs of aging but implied an imbalance of the bodily humours, or humors. It remained paramount for a lady to appear youthful and therefore beautiful to attract the opposite sex in order to secure good marriage. Marriage, after all, was the bargaining chip of the upper classes, in particular, who were forever in pursuit of power, wealth and dynastic influence by means of the institution. In a private letter dating from the early fifteenth century written by a mother to her son on the subject of a prospective new daughter-in-law, the mother notes that, 'I saw her without cosmetics in low heeled shoes so what I saw fits with what I have been told.' A woman was essentially a commodity. The buyer always had to beware of being duped. Clearly a woman had to get her make-up just right not simply for maximum effect but to avoid getting it wrong and spoiling the illusion of youth and beauty entirely, a fault that could cost her dearly in terms of wealth, status and security.

The Handsome Man

In this period men often sported beards. Facial hair was a key distinguishing bodily feature as regards the identification of gender. To keep one's beard in good condition, flower waters could be applied (as they often were to the rest of the hair too) at the barbers, though if a man was wealthy enough he might have servants within his own household who could carry out this task. A man might have his beard dyed, perhaps, to conceal grey but he might do so for other reasons too. For example, men dyed their beards red using saffron and sulphur powder in the reign of Elizabeth I to show their allegiance to the Virgin Queen whose own red hair, also dyed, was such a prominent personal feature. Here we have an early example of appearance in the form of make-up for the purpose of making a political statement. Hygiene products such as teeth cleaners and breath fresheners were used by men as well as women. There were always some men who went much further than basic hygiene and personal grooming of facial hair but the serious trend for men wearing make-up was yet to come.

Make-up and Disease

In this period, as had been the case in the preceding centuries, there was a distinct overlap between what made an individual look beautiful and what made him or her look healthy and by default more attractive. Diseases such as smallpox, the venereal disease syphilis, (also known as the French Pox), and leprosy were rife. Syphilis was almost as dangerous and as widespread as the Black Death had been a century earlier. Without antibiotics to treat these infections, the skin erupted in a rash with open sores and hair loss. Syphilis could even lead to blindness and insanity. Equally, if you survived smallpox, the disease often left marks on the skin. Some foundations such as white lead provided at least a temporary cover-up for the effects of these disfiguring diseases. However, although some might initially see effective results these benefits were often exactly that; short-lived and potentially very harmful.

Cosmetics in Contemporary Literature

This was an age when men still liked to express their opinions on the matter of make-up but at least some women had begun to write down their thoughts and ideas about their own appearance and that of women in general, to record early scientific experiments and to keep and publish books of recipes and other useful household hints. Make-up continued to crop up, as it had done in the Middle Ages, as a topic in conduct books, medical tomes, herbals, cookery books and general household manuals. Conduct or etiquette books, as they were known, were largely aimed at women and set down the rules of expected behaviour, including the care and presentation of one's appearance. Herbals, which concentrated on the treatment of medical ailments, also contained recipes for cosmetics and, by the sixteenth century, had become extremely popular. In fact, Bankes' famous herbal, first published in 1525, was so much admired that it ran to a second edition in only its second year. Cookery books and general household manuals included recipes (or receipts) for powders and perfumes alongside methods for baking pies and cakes and, by so doing, gave a full account to those managing a household of all the information and skills in preparation and organisation they might need. Satirical poetry and essays, as well as plays for the stage, made reference to make-up too. Poems mocked the ugly and the heavily made-up. Contemporary dramatists, including William Shakespeare, made much of the importance of appearance and in plays for the stage humorous catalogues of cosmetic ingredients became a common theatrical device. Matters cosmetic were also discussed in the new alchemical texts, an early form of scientific study in which elite women in particular took a great interest, very often conducting their own experiments.

Books of Secrets

Women and men in the classical world had been credited, correctly or sometimes incorrectly, with specific recipes; remember, for instance, the cure for baldness attributed to Queen Cleopatra by Galen as well as Galen's own innovative recipe for cold cream. In the Renaissance period, recipes ascribed to a particular individual, often a woman of wealth and high status, might be compiled together in a form that became known as a Book of Secrets. These texts are compilations of technical, practical and quasi-scientific instruction, often drawn from the personal experience of the author. Although we might simply refer to these as books of receipts or recipes, instead these were called Books of Secrets because they were written in Latin and their contents were therefore available only to the privileged few who could read or access them. Furthermore, in a practical sense the recipes were not useable by everyone because of the variety, the sheer number, the quantity and the cost of some of the ingredients. Initially at least, there was an element if not exactly of total secrecy, then certainly of exclusivity about these texts. However, with the invention of the printing press, larger-scale publishing reached a growing audience and these Books of Secrets were no longer quite so secret. Versions of them came flooding off the presses in languages other than formal Latin. Elite women compiled recipes for cosmetics that they themselves had apparently found effective, often referring to these as new, unique or their own personal invention. There was a middle-class audience desperate to lap up this information and advice and, in so doing, to emulate these well-to-do women. What had been a secret instead became public knowledge, even if much of it – on account of cost – remained out of the sphere of the less well-off. This endorsement of cosmetic products by individual members of the aristocracy really represents the beginnings of modern advertising.

Although these Books of Secrets are a valuable and fascinating resource, they are not without problems when it comes to interpreting their contents. There are difficulties with translation, for example. Translating the text with the exact nuance, or using the correct name for a plant known locally as something else, can be a challenge for us, and was very likely a challenge for many of those trying to follow the recipes at the time they were written. While we may have more information perhaps in terms of a list of ingredients, a method and descriptions of processes involving decoction (that is, boiling down a liquid to reduce it) distillation or infusion, there are problems with the lack of quantities or gaps in the information. Owing to the sheer variety and the many local variations in respect of the different weights and measures used at the time, even where amounts appear in the instructions, there are difficulties in understanding them. Attempts to recreate cosmetics from this period also run into difficulties, especially when the ingredients themselves cannot be safely handled (as in the case of lead or mercury, for example) or where these ingredients cannot be used for legal reasons – swans are a protected species so swans' fat used in ancient, and in Renaissance make-up cannot be used in any kind of reconstruction of these recipes today.

Alessio Piemontese and his Book of Secrets

The name Alessio Piemontese was almost certainly a pseudonym used by Girilamo Ruscelli (1471–1566), a physician and alchemist living and working in Italy in the late fifteenth and early sixteenth century. His Book of Secrets, first published in 1565 at the very end of his life, purports to recount experiments by the earliest scientific society for which we have any record. This was an organisation based in Naples. Ruscelli's work can certainly be counted as successful. It ran to more than 100 editions and was translated into a large number of different languages. Copies circulated over a long period, from the mid-sixteenth century until the eighteenth century. As this Book of Secrets was so ubiquitous, we cannot fail to conclude that the recipes in it were widely read and, when time and money allowed, widely used. Ruscelli includes cures for bad breath and a soap to wash one's hair to make [it] 'faire'. For skin 'to make the face faire', he recommends bean blossoms - probably castor oil seeds. The Ancient Greek historian Herodotus had suggested using these as a body ointment to soften the skin. Castor oil is still a common ingredient in lipsticks, bath oils and nail polish today. Ruscelli also includes a recipe for what is effectively an early chemical peel, comprising eggs, vinegar, turpentine, sugar-candy, camphor, rock alum (a fine, white potassium-based powder), quicksilver (mercury), lemon juice, tart arum (a salt) and white onion mixed to a paste. He says, 'at night when you go to bedde lay the said composite upon your face neck and breast letting it to drie of itself'. This was then to be left on 'for the space of eight days and although you would think that said composition burned or frayed off the skinne of your face you may not for all that take it off'. This is a highly acidic and corrosive mixture with a powerful odour. Women were expected to suffer for their art.

Isabella Cortese and Her Book of Secrets

Isabella may be one of these wealthy women who put their name directly to a Book of Secrets and by so doing endorse the products contained within it. However, there is some question over whether the book was in fact written by a man under a female pseudonym. If we take what we have in terms of the evidence at face value, then all we know about Isabella is that she was, according to her own work, a woman who practised alchemy, the precursor of modern chemistry, mixed with a little philosophy and magic. The alchemists' main aim was to turn base metals into gold. However, experiments were carried out into the production of other materials and the book is no doubt the result of her (or maybe his) personal experiments over a number of years. Cortese's three-volume work ran to twelve editions between 1561 and 1677.

The full title of the work is *The Secrets of Signora Isabella Cortese in which are included mineral man-made and alchemical things and many things concerning the art of perfumery suitable for any lady*. While there are many interesting topics covered in the text, including how to dye gloves yellow and perhaps rather more surprisingly how to make invisible ink, it is in the third volume of the work that the said Isabella concentrates on how to make cosmetics and perfumes. She (or perhaps he) recommends the following under the heading 'A beauty water for the Face': 'Take lemons and dried beans and combine in white wine; add honey, egg, and goat's milk, and distil it all together; and this water will make the face beautiful.'

Thankfully there is nothing harmful here. In fact, the mixture consists of some straightforward ingredients that could be found in many kitchens then and now. However, the book also includes the following rather more complex recipe for a good complexion:

Take two pigeons with white feathers and feed them on pine nuts for eight, or rather fifteen, days; then butcher them and throw away the head, feet, and guts; put [the rest] in an alembic and distil with half a loaf of sweetened bread and four ounces of true silver, three gold ducats, four heels of white bread that has been left to soften in goat's milk for six days ... distil all of this over low heat, and it will produce a most perfect water to give colour to a pale complexion.

Some recipes, like this one, were based on what we would call sympathetic magic, that is, ritual where there is some correlation, whether real or symbolic, between the objects used and the person or persons one intends to influence. Note that the pigeons in the recipe quoted above must have white feathers. This is an example of magical belief in the transference of colour from one thing to another. The white of the bird's feathers was believed to become a mixture that would produce a pale complexion. Another example of this element of magic is evident in Isabella's recipe for maintaining the hands in good condition. She recommends 'white hen water for making hands beautiful fresh and maintaining youth'. Again note the correlation between the white hen and the white hands. The magic or superstition that is clearly an important element of these recipes seems to be a step backward from the medieval text, the *Trotula Minor* which excludes these elements. However we have to remember that the Trotula was rather the exception to the rule as far as this was concerned.

The Medici Family

Caterina Sforza (1463–1509) was not only the countess of the cities of Forli and Imola but also a member of the affluent and extremely influential Medici family whose power base was the fashionable city of Florence. While it goes without saying that she was a woman of some considerable social standing, Caterina was also an important figure in the development of cosmetics. There is a Book of Secrets attributed to her known as the *Experimenti*. The text included 192 cosmetic recipes for the face, skin, hair, teeth, and gums. The ingredients in her recipes include camphor, egg whites, rose water, white lead, alum, quicksilver, lye (otherwise known as sodium hydroxide or to put it more simply caustic soda), arsenic, ivy resin and ants' eggs. She recommends mint and rosemary as breath fresheners and the use of animal bones to clean around one's teeth. Quicksilver, lye and white lead are all highly corrosive and poisonous. Caterina includes toilet waters and many recipes to care for the skin and repair skin damage, some of which could easily have been caused by some of the recipes she herself quotes. Men as well as women asked her for advice. Caterina Sforza's knowledge of the ingredients of her cosmetics was soundly based, as it was on her own alchemical experiments. She retains her mystique and selling power to this day, appearing in twentieth century computer games and Japanese manga comics.

Don Antonio de Medici (1576–1621), although perhaps not a prominent character in terms of economic or political standing, did play an important role in respect of make-up, leaving for future generations a manuscript that details a long list of ingredients that were often in common use at this time. His particular interest seems to have been in skin care and products to whiten the complexion. He recommends everything from the safe, and potentially effective, to the downright dangerous. The dangerous such as white lead, quicksilver and rock alum feature as usual, as do the safe options of lemon juice, goat's milk and even sugar. Some of his other suggestions might not be exactly dangerous in a chemical sense but could damage the skin, cutting or bruising its surface: pieces of porcelain vases used to clear the skin for example. Other skin care products in this list involved crushing the ingredients to a powder. According to Don Antonio 'snails make the face shiny soft and beautiful and the ones without the shells are the best but must be washed well ... those with the shells have to be well crushed.' He also recommends white seashells to make skin white and beautiful. They are used in powdered form or dissolved in lemon juice.

A *Spanish Cookery Book*

A sixteenth century Spanish cookbook known as the *Manual de Mugeres* is typical of a contemporary kitchen recipe book in that it contains recipes that range from how to make a chorizo sausage to washes for the face. The manual is written in the vernacular, an indication that at every level of society there was interest in this subject matter and a demand for wider dissemination of knowledge, moving away from the more formal texts written in Latin. These compilations of recipes, which included cosmetics alongside and sometimes interchangeable with medicines, but also with cookery and cleaning preparations, were plentiful from mid-sixteenth century right up until the eighteenth century. While books like this one were literally 'how to' books, they were not just practical manuals, as they also showed a philosophical and quasi-scientific or alchemic side, and sometimes made personal references to the women who used this make-up to promote the use of particular products; for example, excellent beauty water used by the D of C, or beauty water for the face by Madam G. The exact identity of these individuals may be unknown to us, but it is likely that the women referred to were known to contemporary readers.

Herbals

The work of writers such as Pliny the Elder (AD 23–AD 79) and Greek writer Dioscorides (who died in AD 90), are the precursors of the early modern herbal. While the herbals that circulated in the Middle Ages mostly dealt with herbs for culinary or medicinal purposes, the later herbals from the latter half of the fifteenth and into the sixteenth centuries began to include more recipes for cosmetics. The botanist William Turner's herbal, published in three volumes between the years 1551 and 1568, notes some cosmetic recipes – albeit with a thinly veiled criticism of beauty treatments in general. According to Turner, marigolds may be of use to those who are not satisfied with their own hair colour (that is, as a source of hair dye), while cowslip mixed with white wine can beautify the complexion for women 'to make themselves faire in the eyes of the world rather than the eyes of God whom they are not afraid to offend'.

The Condemnation of Cosmetics

There was still plenty of criticism of women (and men) who used cosmetics – and not only in herbals such as the work of William Turner quoted above. Disapproval was especially reserved for those who were perceived as using these products to excess, or perhaps in an attempt to conceal their age or true identity. Some authors, especially those who were members of the Church hierarchy, were consistent in their condemnation of cosmetics regardless of how much, or how little, might have been applied. In Italy, disapproval of cosmetics began to take a very physical and rather sinister form. In what became known as the Bonfires of the Vanities, things associated with excess such as books in which make-up was the subject matter and objects used in the adornment of the body, such as combs and mirrors, were ritually burnt. The largest of these bonfires took place in Florence on 7 February 1497 at the behest of the powerful Dominican priest Savonarola. The extent to which churchmen felt it necessary to condemn make-up and to take the kind of action that Savonarola thought expedient may be an indication not only of the strength of feeling of the Church in relation to make-up but also testament to the widespread use of these beauty products. It was not only the Church that disapproved of cosmetics. The words quoted at the beginning of this chapter taken from a work by Giovanni Della Casa (1503–1556), a Florentine poet, diplomat and writer on matters of etiquette, also express criticism. However, his objection is to men wearing make-up. He does not comment on whether or not women should do so.

There were grounds upon which this dislike of make-up might be considered reasonable when seen through the eyes of contemporary Renaissance society. In the first place, many cosmetics, especially those at the more expensive end of the market, were imported and, on account of their cost, tended to create an economic imbalance between exports and imports. Secondly, beauty products promoted vanity, a sin and contrary to the teachings of the Church. Thirdly, many of these products were simply bad for the person using them, to the point of being potentially fatal. Finally, there were those who decried the confusion caused in identifying a person's ethnic identity on account of the make-up they wore. The English satirist Stephen Gosson (1554–1613) for example, wrote 'these painted faces which they wear can any tell from whence they come?' The English historian and topographer William Camden (1551–1623) went so far as to associate the use of cosmetics with barbarous peoples. Perhaps the strongest accusation levelled against the use of cosmetics was the opportunity for deceit that these products offered the individual. The idea of cosmetics as a tool in the art of deception had been widely expressed from classical times and the connotation had stuck. In a cruel and vivid analogy, the sixteenth century pamphleteer Joseph Swetnam describes the woman who paints herself as 'like the spider which weaves a fine web to land the flie', the victim in this case being the unsuspecting man.

However, despite the prevalence of such strong criticism, a fashion for books that offered advice and instruction emerged as an alternative. This trend combined with the fact that at least some of the texts that mention make-up were compiled by women themselves, means that by the sixteenth century, we no longer have to extrapolate information, to the same extent, from evidence that is strongly weighted against the use of cosmetics. Besides being able to read a number of texts, albeit a relatively small number attributed to women, we have men finding reasons to write more positively about this subject. These less-critical texts are coupled with an enthusiasm for the actual wearing of make-up, by women in particular. Men who wore cosmetics were less likely to get this new-found good press.

Skin Care

While getting rid of the physical vestiges of disease such as pockmarks was important, in accordance with both the fashion and religious belief of the day, it was also essential to eliminate or disguise other skin blemishes such as freckles. Freckles were believed to be the devil's marks. According to Sir Hugh Plat (1552–1608), an English writer and inventor who enthusiastically collected information on a wide variety of topics, 'To take away the freckles in the face, wash your face in the wane of the moon with a spunge morninge evening with the distilled water of elder leaves letting the same dey into the skinne. Your water must be distilled'. Plat claimed to have acquired this recipe from a traveller who, in turn, claimed that this recipe had worked for him. Note the strong element of superstition contained within the instructions. The method seems to have as much to do with magic and pagan rituals as any scientific merit and though the elder leaves are now believed have some anti-inflammatory properties, the procedure was hardly likely to remove any freckles. Culpepper in his well-known herbal suggests cowslips, a crop sold in bunches, for medicinal and beauty purposes, as well as a wine ingredient. These flowers, he alleged; 'an ointment being made with them taketh away spots and wrinkles of the skin sunburnings and freckles and promotes beauty'. Johann Jacob Wecker (1528–1586) gives us the following recipe in his *Eighteen Books of the Secrets of Art & Nature being the Summe and Substance of Natural Philosophy specifically intended for this purpose*: 'For Freckles of the face. Take Rosewater juice of Lemons, each eight ounces Sublimate two drams, four whites of Eggs, mix them all well, then set it in the sun for eight days, and keep it for your use.' A dram or drachm was an apothecary's measure; one ounce equals eight drachms. Women and men washed their faces not with soap but with an exfoliating mixture of flour and seeds. The Spanish cookbook the *Manual de Mugeres* recommends a variety of beans and seeds including kidney beans, lupin seeds and white radish seeds, mixed together. These were ground and sifted to make what would have been to all intents and purposes, a reasonably effective exfoliating cleanser. This was probably a relatively cheap product too, as beans and seeds such as these were very much part of the everyday diet of the poor. There was a tradition of including lupin seeds in skin care, stretching back to ancient times. Note that lupin seeds were an important ingredient in the extant face pack recipes of the Roman poet Ovid. Fruit and flower waters also softened and cleansed the skin. Bankes' herbal suggests rosemary mixed with white wine to improve the complexion. Soliman's water, a face cleanser, is a good example not only of an early cosmetic ascribed a 'brand name' if you like, but also of a cosmetic that would have appeared to have worked initially but could eventually have lead to permanent skin damage. A mixture of mercury, sulphur and turpentine, Soliman's water was a corrosive concoction that would certainly get rid of spots in the short term but did so simply by removing the top layer of skin. Soliman's water is an example of an early, and highly dangerous, chemical peel. Aside from the fact that its application in the longer term could result in skin damage, this product could also cause receding gums and, as a result, loosen teeth, and might finally cause poisoning and death. The name Soliman's water suggests that this product may have come to Europe from the East, though its precise origins remain a mystery; the name may simply be intended to conjure up a sense of exoticism and therefore make this more desirable and more marketable. Oil of vitriol or sulphuric acid, a highly corrosive product, was also used in skin care and again would have caused long-term damage.

A book entitled *The Worth of Women*, and subtitled 'wherein is clearly revealed their nobility and their superiority to men', written under the pseudonym of Moderata Fonte (believed to have been a respectable Venetian woman), takes the form of a dialogue between seven Venetian noblewomen (1592) and contains the following skin care recipe; 'I've heard said Cornelia that if you boil down a calf's foot for forty days the liquid can get rid of wrinkles and make your skin as smooth as that of a girl of fifteen.'

In fact this recipe appears much earlier (in the first century AD to be precise) in Pliny the Elder's Natural Histories. Renaissance scholars, who were not only fascinated by these ancient texts but busily translating them, would no doubt have discovered this information and considered it useful wisdom from the ancient world – the work of Pliny the Elder, though it would fall out of favour in later centuries, was particularly popular at this time. Bear's grease was another cosmetic popular in Roman times that was applied to the face in the fifteenth and sixteenth centuries to soften the skin. Rosewater was popular as a skin softener and toner too, well known even at this early date for its anti-inflammatory qualities. Milk, an emollient or softener, could be effective when applied to the skin and had an even longer history going back to the days of Queen Cleopatra. Both milk and rosewater were not only safe and effective but were certainly more pleasant smelling solution to skin problems than Soliman's water, for example, although neither would have removed the more deep-seated scars of a disease like smallpox.

Hand Creams

A lady's hands needed special attention. They were often the first part of a prospective wife's anatomy that her future husband might see or touch, perhaps greeting her on an initial meeting. Hands could be cited legitimately as an attractive feature at an early stage in any courtship. Ladies' hands, when not inside gloves, might also be on show to the public in general so it was important that they made a good first impression. A woman of some social standing should have hands that were both soft and paper white. Rough red hands were the hands of those involved in manual labour; that is, the lower classes. The sixteenth century Spanish cookbook the *Manual de Mugeres* recommends the following preparation for softening the hands:

> Take marrow from six sheep and the top of the skulls from their heads and a loaf of kid tallow of the size of an *excudilla* (a bowl) and mix it all together. Melt and wash it with crude water and after with rose water and then with lemon juice. Then add a little of this juice together with the water from fresh argol (a form of tartar formed in wine casks from grape sediment) and mix it well. And after it has been washed well add with it two ounces of bitter almond oil and four ounces of opium poppy oil. And stir everything together. And once it is well mixed keep in various bottles.

Here we are beginning to get the occasional mention of weights and measures in recipes. To me, it seems likely that producing this at home would take some practised skill to get the mixture right, as well as assuming easy access to a good number of livestock. However, the fact that the text states that this mixture can be stored, and therefore made in bulk, is certainly a plus point. The almond oil the mixture contains would be effective in softening skin. Indeed it is still used today for this purpose, while lemon juice can not only freshen and cleanse but also has the potential to whiten skin. Isabella Cortese in her (or indeed his) Book of Secrets recommends the following treatment for hands;

> take some lemon juice and the same quantity of perfumed water and place it on the fire to boil. While this is boiling pour in some powdered almond skins and stir turning it into soap.

Wash your hands with it and it will make your hands soft white and beautiful.

Although the measurements are not precise, there are at least guidelines to follow – in this case, reference to equal quantities. This recipe is also less complex than many in terms of preparation and the number of ingredients. However, the instructions suggest that this was a hand cream made in much smaller amounts. The ingredients themselves are, in some cases, the same as those in the previous recipe taken from the Spanish cookbook and this cosmetic might effect the desired result: a pale smooth skin. In his herbal Gerard recommends oil of almonds to make 'smooth the hands and face of delicate persons and cleanseth the skin form all spots and pimples'. Almond oil is a simple and effective moisturiser that is still readily available at cosmetic counters today.

Foundations and Powders

White lead continued to be a favourite foundation despite the known risks to the skin and the potential damage to the internal organs, and the knowledge that regular contact with it and that the application of white lead could even lead to mental confusion, muscle paralysis, poisoning, and even death. The dangers of handling white lead, never mind actually applying it directly onto the skin and wearing it over the day, are remarked upon by contemporary artists who used this substance to paint portraits and scenery for the stage. Lomazzo (1538–1592) an Italian painter and writer on the theory of art in his *Tracte Containing the Artes of Curious Paintinge Carvinge and Buildinge* remarks,

The ceruse or white lead which women use to better their complexion is made of lead and vinegar; which mixture is naturally a great drier; and it is used by chirurgions (an archaic spelling of the word surgeons) to drie up moiste sores. So that those women who use it about their faces do quickly become withered and gray headed because this doth so mightily drie up the natural moisture of their flesh.

White lead would, in later years, be used by cabinetmakers to treat wood (limed oak) and seal porous wood against insect infestation. This gives us some idea of its potency. Despite these dangers, lead remained popular and the wealthy sought out the best quality product available. The best white lead on sale at this time was known as Spirits of Saturn, or Venetian ceruse. Venetian ceruse was made from pure white lead unadulterated by any substitute that was often added to white lead to eke it out. Scented starch was a much safer product, though not as highly regarded in terms of its effectiveness. Ground alabaster could also create a very desirable porcelain look. Powdered borax (a mild alkali), still used in face creams and other cosmetic products today, was another safe alternative to white lead on the market at this time. Pale translucent skin allowed veins to stand out or, if they didn't stand out enough, these could be painted onto the skin. Blue veins suggested royal blood and had its origin in stories in which the Spanish royals compared themselves with the conquered Moors.

Make-up could be sealed with an application of egg white. This not only acted as a fixative but also gave a much-admired glazed finish. However, the veneer also made it virtually impossible to express emotion – to smile or frown, for example. The philosopher Alessandro Piccolomini (1508–1578) in his *Dialogue of the Fair Perfectioning of Ladies* describes this problem in detail:

So handsomely had she covered her face that I promise you her eyes seemed those of another woman; for the cold had made her complexion a ghastly yellow like lead and dried plastering so that the poor woman had to stand stiffly and not turn her head but with her whole body for fear the mask should split.

Rouge

Colour could be added to the cheeks by applying red plant dyes extracted from the roots of herbs such as madder or alkanet. Cochineal was also an option in the late fifteenth and sixteenth centuries. This was sometimes mixed with talcum powder and rosewater for ease of application. Red ochre continued to be used on the cheeks, as it had been from prehistoric times. Henry Peacham (1546–1634), an English poet and writer, remarked that; 'for a penny a chambermaid may buy as much red ochre as serve seven years for the painting of her cheeks'. No doubt this is an exaggeration, but clearly red ochre was not expensive rouge in the early modern period and therefore available to all, even those, like the chambermaid, on the lowest rungs of the employment ladder. The wealthier, in keeping with their status, would want to use something else entirely. Different shades of red were more or less expensive depending on what they were made from. Vermillion, a very intense and bright shade of red, what we might describe as scarlet, was made from ground powdered cinnabar and, being particularly highly regarded and in much demand, vermillion was expensive to buy. Therefore to be seen in public wearing this immediately gave out a message of substantial wealth and status. However vermillion was extremely poisonous so expressing one's wealth in this way was fraught with danger to a lady's health. Rock alum could be rubbed on the skin to heigthen the complexion and add colour. In fact, all this was doing, as Lomazzo put it, was causing 'hurt to the face …oner droppe thereof being put upon the skinne, burneth, shriveth and parcheth with divers other inconveniences like loosing the teeth'. This was hardly the way to create a healthy and attractive appearance.

Hair

In Federico Luigini's *Book of the Beautiful Woman* (1554), the author imagines, in his dreams, that he and his friends spend an evening 'taking up brushes and colour' to paint the ideal woman. He says,

> I desire to take first her hair: for that me thinks is more important to her beauty than any of her other charms seeing as without it she would be as a garden without flowers or a ring without jewels ... Tresses therefore must adorn our lady and in colour they shall be like unto clear shining gold.

Leaving aside the colour for the moment, keeping one's hair in good order was a sign of an upright and moral lifestyle. The fashion for thick hair was a sign not only of style and glamour and an important position in society, but also of good health. Baldness was one of the most visible symptoms of syphilis. The use of lead-based cosmetics could result in hair loss too. Others suffered from premature baldness unrelated to disease. Some products promised to thicken, and at the same time pleasantly perfume, the hair though we might justifiably doubt the merits of the following recipe which comes from our Spanish cookbook in this respect:

> Whoever desires to have their hair grow a lot to make the head smell very good should get used to combing the hair with vulture grease in the sun.

The wording of the text itself implies that the resulting scent is an acquired taste. Between washes, perfumed bran was used as a dry shampoo. Baldness, whatever the reason, could of course be remedied by donning a wig.

According to Philip Stubbes, a sixteenth century pamphleteer, in his diatribe against excessive attention to the appearance entitled

The Anatomies of Abuses (1583) some men when visiting the barbers had

> ...the haire of the nostrils cut away and everything done in order comely to behold ... too shall have also your orient perfumes for your nose, your fragrant waters for your face wherewith you shall be all to besprinkled: your musick again and pleasant harmony shall sound in your ears and all though tickle the same with vaine delight and in the end your choice shall be brushed and 'god be with you gentleman'!

Blonde was still the favourite shade for women, at least as in contemporary literature and art. According to Firenzuola 'A lady's hair should be fine and fair. In the similitude now of gold, now of honey, and now of the shining rays of the sun'. Indeed, Firenzuola's description of the ideal colour for a lady's hair is typically classical in style, comparing as it does her locks with elements of the natural world. In *The Book of Natural Magick* by the scientist and scholar Giambattista della Porta published in 1584, there are a number of recipes for blonde hair dyes including this one:

> To make the hair yellow. Thus, they put into a common lye the citron pills, oranges, quinces, barley straw, dried lupines feny-greac, broom flowers and tartar coloured a good quantity. And let them there lie and steep to wash their hair with.

Alexis of Piedmontese (aka Ruscelli) in his Book of Secrets refers to a soap used to wash hair to make it thick and fair and to achieve the desired red-blonde effect. He recommends dyes such as saffron, turmeric or rhubarb. The latter is strong but still recommended as a natural hair dye. More dangerous was lye, a sort of caustic soda. What is described in these two recipes, and others that date from this period, as a wash or a soap are, in fact, dyes for the hair. Horse urine or alternatively a mixture of juice and saffron could be applied to tint one's hair blonde too. Powdering hair with gold dust might achieve a blonde or at least a lightening effect. I am struck by the numerous ingredients in many of these recipes as well as in the time taken to prepare them, which often ran to days or even weeks. I wonder too how these products were stored, as surely they must have been, as these dyes were prepared in such large quantities. Another explanation might be that all the women of the household used this dye at once. What is not in doubt is that many women set aside time and made considerable efforts to make their hair look good. Philip Stubbes, who roundly condemns cosmetics in his writing, claims women go to extraordinary lengths to secure blonde locks,

> They are not simply content with their owne haire, but buy other heyre, dying of what colour they list themselves; and if there be any poore woman that hath faire haire these nice dames will not rest, till they have bought it. Or if any children have faire haire, they will entice them into a secrete place and for a penie or two, they will cut off their haire.

For bleaching hair Giovanni Marinello, an Italian physician and gynaecologist, writing in his book *Beautification of the Ladies*, suggests the following; 'take the fried dregs of white wine and chop them into olive oil. Comb this through your hair while sitting in the sun'. This instruction, he says, is in response to the demands for information on how to care for hair from his clients. The text and its author also reflect the continued close association between make-up and medicine. In order to protect one's complexion from the sun while bleaching one's hair at the same time, a woman donned a Solana, a wide-brimmed straw hat with the hole in the crown. Cesar Vecellio, an artist working in Venice towards the end of the sixteenth century, notes that sitting in the sun to bleach one's hair was common practice among the well-to-do ladies of that fashionable city: He gives such detail on this that is easy to create a picture of it in the mind's eye: 'It is customary in Venice', he says, 'to erect square open loggias onto houses ... there the greater part of the women of Venice devotes themselves intensely to the art of dying their hair blond employing different kinds of washes ands rinses especially devised for this purpose ... wearing to protect themselves from the sun a lightweight straw hat called a Solana with a hole in the top through which they pull their hair. The women wet their locks with small sponges attached to a slender stick while admiring themselves in a mirror.' This sounds rather like touching up the roots.

Not all hair dyes were intended to lighten hair. Combs, known as black lead combs, were dipped in black lead to restore dark hair and to cover any grey. These may also have been kept in lead boxes. In presenting an indication of one's overall health and constitution, one's hair should match one's complexion. In his *Ninth Book of Natural Magic* under the heading 'how to dye the hair red' Della Porta explains that this is precisely the reason why a man or woman choose red. He says this is, 'because there are many men and women that have ruddy complexions and have their hair of their heads and beards red which should they make yellow coloured they would not agree with their complexions'. To make the hair red, Isabella Cortese recommends:

six ounces of walnut oil three ounces of white honey and three ounces of burnt tartar quenched in a glass of white wine leave for twenty-four hours so that wine absorbs the substance of the tartar then take the wine with the honey and put into a glazed pot with some grains of burnt cumin and the said oil, Cook until the honey burns and the wine has completely evaporated strain and conserve the oil in a flask. When you have your hair dressed anoint the comb with the salad oil and comb the hair in the sun and the oil will make it red.

Hugh Plat suggests the following alternative:

How to colour the head or beard into a chestnut colour in half an hour. Take one part of lead calcined with sulphur and one parte of quicke lime temper them somewhat thin with water lay upon the hair chafing it well in and let it dry one quarter of an houre or thereabout then wash the same off with faire water divers times and lastly with soap and water and it will it will be a verie natural hair colour. The longer it lyeth on the hair the browner it groweth this coloureth not the flesh at all and yety it lasteth verie long in the hair.

This is just what we might want from a modern hair colorant though without having to resort to dangerous ingredients such as, lead, sulphur and quicklime.

Hair Removal

Other things unfortunately diminish your charms making your skin fetid and stinking. One of these things is body hair.
Giovanni Marinello, *Gli Ornamenti delle donne*

For women a hairless body was *de rigueur* and, just as had been the case in ancient and medieval times, hair removal was practised for hygiene purposes as well as to enhance one's overall attractiveness. Unlike the classical period but in accordance with a trend that began in the Middle Ages, women also depilated their forehead and the temples as well as the more usual places. A high forehead was considered beautiful though whether this was necessitated by the corrosive nature of some of the face creams and foundations that eat away the hair or whether the fashion itself came first remains a moot point. Caterina Sforza records nine recipes for the removal of hair including this one:

> Take 2 ounces of quicklime, 1 ounce of arsenic, and as much rock alum as you could fit in a chestnut, and grind it all together in a powder very well, then knead with gold ... paste it where you want the hairs to fall out. Leave it for the time it takes to say two 'Our Fathers' then wash it off.

As ever, in the case of many of these early depilatories, the ingredients are dangerous to the extent of being poisonous and made from caustic substances such as quicklime or arsenic. Della Porta mentions the following recipe under the heading 'A common depilatory':

> It consists of quicklime four parts made into powder orpiment one part. Try with a hen feather when that is made bare with it, it is boiled. Take heed not to boil it too much or that it stays not too long upon your skin for it will burn. But if it chance to burn your skin take populeum and oil of roses or violets and anoint the place and the pain will be gone.

Clearly the writer was aware of the potential dangers of this corrosive mixture and therefore advises the user to be ready with a remedy, albeit one which would seem to have little chance of relieving the pain, damage or discomfort. As well as depilatories that temporarily removed any unwanted body hair, Della Porta included recipes for concoctions that allegedly encouraged hair to grow more slowly and even treatments that promised to stop unwanted hair growing again altogether. He suggests an application oil of henbane or hemlock or, apparently for men in particular, a mixture of ant's eggs, red orpiment, red volcanic rock (containing arsenic) and ivy gum mixed with vinegar to slow down the re-growth of unwanted hair. Under the heading 'so that the hair should never grow again' Della Porta prescribes saltpetre in water, oil of brimstone (a sulphurous mineral) or vitriol (known today as sulphuric acid).

Lips, Teeth and Gums

Lip colour was fashionable. This consisted of ground alabaster or Plaster of Paris mixed with alkanet or cochineal for colour. The finished product looked rather like a wax crayon. Queen Elizabeth is known to have worn lipstick made from cochineal, gum Arabic, egg white and fig milk.

The desire for white teeth is not a modern phenomenon. Those who could afford it endeavoured to keep their teeth clean and white chiefly to avoid the connotations of poverty and disease associated with black teeth. Both men and women used pumice stone or cuttlefish bone to remove black stains caused by syphilis but because this was somewhat abrasive, the practice was inclined to remove the tooth enamel too. White and even pastel enamels could be painted on at a price: anything was acceptable, it seems, as long as it was not black. However, even the wealthy struggled to keep their teeth in good order. Isabella of Aragon, the Duchess of Milan and Bari (1470–1524) and the daughter of King Alphonso of Spain, was known to have teeth that were in poor condition Interestingly she was rumoured to be the subject of Da Vinci's famous painting, the *Mona Lisa*. If this theory is correct, it may explain the *Mona Lisa's* enigmatic expression –a feature often commented on. Like the *Mona Lisa*, Isabella was reluctant to smile, not wishing to expose her bad teeth to view. Mouth and teeth preparations including pastilles to chew were used to counteract bad breath. There were also mixtures for tightening the teeth and gums to help prevent the loss of teeth. The English writer and inventor Sir Hugh Plat (1552–1608), in his popular work *Delights for Ladies,* recommends the following treatment: 'To keepe the teeth both white and sound. Take a quart of honey as much vinegar and halfe so much white wine, boyle them together and wash your teeth therewith now and then'.

Cosmetics for the Bust

Firenzuola states that the 'bosom must be white' and William Horman (1440 –1535) the headmaster at Eton, also makes this observation remarking that '[Women] whyte theyr face, necke and pappis with cerusse'. Certainly, the trend for low-cut dresses left much of the shoulders and bust exposed. Fashion dictated that any skin open to view should have the same pale white and unblemished appearance as one's complexion. This meant applying whatever foundation a lady was wearing, whether dangerous white lead or a safer chalk-based material, had also to be applied on the neck and décolletage. Courtesans in this period applied ivy oil and rose oil with camphor to improve their bustline. While the camphor may be cooling it has, as we all know when using it to treat a cold, a very strong smell; there is nothing to suggest it would have had any effect in shaping or firming the bust. However, ivy oil is both antibacterial and soothing, while rose oil might have counteracted the pungent smell of the camphor, although the mixture could equally be described as potentially overpowering. According to the journal of the Ambassador to King Henry IV of France, on meeting Queen Elizabeth,

> She kept the front of her dress open and one could see the whole of her bosom and passing low and often she would open the front of the robe with her hands as if she was too hot

... her bosom is somewhat wrinkled ... but lower down her flesh is exceeding white and delicate so far as one could see.

Elizabeth was not a young woman when this encounter took place so to modern tastes at least, this is all rather shocking in its detail.

Eyes and Eyebrows

Applying eye make up was not part of the lady's toilette in this period. However putting drops of belladonna extract (also known as deadly nightshade) to give the effect of large sparkling eyes was still popular. Although eye make was not worn, women (but not most men) did pay attention to the shape and condition of their eyebrows. Castiglione in his *Book of the Courtier* describes women 'painfully plucking their eyebrows and their forehead and using all those little tricks and suffering all those little agonies which you ladies imagine that men know nothing but which they know only too well'. Della Porta mentions preparations to dye one's eyebrows with burnt black earth or ox bone mixed with soot.

Drama: Face Painting on Stage and Off...

Shakespeare puts the following words into the mouth of the eponymous character in his play *Hamlet* when he addresses Ophelia, 'God has given you one face and you make yourself another'. In fact, this was true both on the stage and off it and Shakespeare knew this only too well. In the early modern world, dramatists were very aware of visual impact of their productions. Theatre created a spectacle in a number of different ways. Attending a play was about understanding the action on the stage through listening to the dialogue but also by picking up on the visual signals offered by the characters by means of their costumes, gestures and expressions. Stage make-up was usually applied thickly to accentuate the actors expression and, by so doing, assist the audience in their interpretation of a given character and his or her part in the drama. However, it was not only actors but the audience who were the spectacle at a theatre performance. While the action on the stage was being viewed, the elite members of the audience were also there to be looked at. They sported their best clothes, headgear and, of course, make-up on these occasions for others to notice and admire.

On stage, young men played the female parts as women were not allowed to appear. Instead of using expensive white lead or ceruse to simulate a feminine pale complexion, this was reproduced for the stage more cheaply by applying powdered hog's bones mixed with poppy oil. For a performance of a play with an element of magic, for example Shakespeare's *A Midsummer's Nights Dream*, crushed pearls or silver might be added to the actor's make-up to give off an ethereal shimmer appropriate to the setting and the storyline. Scene painters continued to paint the faces of the actors with the same materials they used for the scenery and backdrops, as they had done in medieval times.

In contemporary drama the painted face could both attract and repel and aside from make-up being an expected part of the actors tool box, we find that there are many references in contemporary drama to make-up and its application bound into the action of the drama itself. Satirical cataloguing of ingredients was not uncommon. Indeed the scene in *Macbeth* where the witches add ingredients to their cauldron is, in effect, a parody of a cosmetic recipe, an allusion that would have been easily understood by a contemporary audience. Cosmetics were a feature of comedy and satire as well as serious drama. In *A Humorous Day's Mirth*, a comedy by playwright George Chapman first performed in 1597, the female character is compared to a piece of parchment:

She reads over her face every morning and sometimes blots out pale and writes red. She thinks she is faire though many times her opinion goes alone ... she is hid away all but her face and that is hanged about with toyes and devices like the signe of a tavern to draw strangers.

The woman's face is artificially contrived, painted very likely with the same preparations that would have been used to paint a sign. The clientele of the tavern was not salubrious. The woman who wears make-up is still being stereotyped as a harlot or woman of loose morals.

Royal ladies: Catherine de Medici

Catherine became Queen of France when she married Henry II in 1533. As well as exotic foodstuffs, she brought with her from her native Italy her knowledge of make-up and fashions in cosmetics. Soon the French court was enjoying these new trends. Catherine's influence helped France become a centre of perfume and cosmetic production. Flowers were produced in market gardens on a grand scale, especially in the south of France, for their scent and made into perfumes.

The raw ingredients also became ingredients in scented ointments, creams and toilet waters. Catherine de Medici's personal perfumer, brought with her from Italy, was named Rene de Florentin by the French court. A skilled alchemist, he had a laboratory in the Louvre in Paris, accessible by a secret passageway to none but Catherine herself. He was crucially important to her politically, as well as in respect of her social position. The secrecy that surrounded the ingredients that he used in his perfumes and scented ointments led to suggestions that he poisoned certain individuals at the queen's request.

Royal Ladies: Elizabeth I

At the English court, the Virgin Queen, Elizabeth I, used cosmetics extensively, especially as she grew older, setting a trend for doing so at least within court circles. In her youth, Elizabeth probably did have the porcelain pale complexion that tends to accompany naturally red hair. However, having suffered from smallpox as a very young woman, she used heavy make-up to cover the damage done to her skin by the disease. Over the years, her use of products containing white lead, mercury and arsenic took their toll so that by the end of her life her real visage is believed to have been concealed under as much as an inch-and-a-half of heavy make-up. There was considerable interest in Elizabeth's health. Her appearance was particularly important because not only was her health believed to be accurately reflected in her appearance, but her physical condition also became a metaphor for the health of the nation as a whole. While many today watch the comings and goings of the royal family, showing an interest in what they wear and how they look, Elizabeth's court considered her appearance to be of the utmost importance to the nation. The queen effectively used make-up to promote herself, concealing her blemishes under an increasingly thick layer of lead. Her portraits also concealed the truth. This would never have been questioned as it was in no way unusual for idealism to win over realism in portraiture, especially when the subject was famous or important in some way. However, one recently discovered portrait believed to be of Queen Elizabeth painted by the Flemish artist Marcus Gheeraerts, (1561–1636) whose work was sought after at the English court, appears to be somewhat more honest. The ravages of age including lines and wrinkles are clearly evident in this work making it hard to imagine that the queen would have wanted such an image on public view.

Elizabeth would appear to have had double standards in that while she was quite happy to wear make-up, she was less keen on others doing so. Indeed the queen decreed that 'any woman who through the use of false hair, Spanish hair pads, make-up, false hips, steel busks, panniers, high heeled shoes or other devices leads a subject of her majesty into marriage shall be punished with the penalties of witchcraft.' Despite Elizabeth's protestations make-up and the art of looking good was big business in England. So much so that elite women in other parts of Europe might request desirable cosmetics from England for their use. For example, Esperanza Malchi, agent of the Sultana of Constantinople, writes to Queen Elizabeth saying:

> On account of your majesty being a woman I can without embarrassment employ you with this notice which is that there are to be found in your kingdom rare distilled waters of every kind for the face and odiferous oils for the hands Your majesty would favour me by sending some of these by hand for this most serene queen.

Note that Esperanza does not wish these valuable products to pass through any other hands on the way to her mistress. There is still an element of secrecy around the best cosmetics used by the most important people at this time.

Royal Ladies: Lucrezia Borgia

The infamous Lucrezia Borgia (1480–1519) the daughter of Pope Alexander VI and a member of yet another famous and powerful Italian family may, or may not, have been a natural blonde. Paintings certainly portray her as fair haired. Another tangible and rather intriguing clue to her hair colouring is sadly just out of our reach. I refer to a lock of Lucrezia's hair given to one Pietro Bembo, probably as a love token and now stored in the Ambrosiana library in Milan. From around 1685 the lock of hair was kept wrapped inside one of Lucrezia's letters.

However, in the eighteenth century Lord Byron tried and failed to get his hands on it and steal it away. In the 1930s, the library's Board of Fellows decided to keep the lock safely sealed inside a decorative reliquary made especially for this purpose by the jeweller Alfredo Ravasco. No analysis of the hair sample has ever been undertaken. While blonde was certainly a fashionable colour, the piece of hair that could give us some answers is just out of reach.

Miscellaneous Recipes
From the Elixirs of Nostradamus: how to introduce gold highlights into your hair.

> Take a pound of finely pulverized beech wood shaving, half a pound of box wood shavings, four ounces of fresh liquorice, a similar amount of swallowwort and yellow poppy seeds two ounces of the leaves and flowers of glacus, a herb which grows in Syria and is akin to the poppy, half an ounce of saffron and half a pound of paste made from finely ground wheat flour... [a description of a long drawn out method follows] and... within three or four days the hair will look as yellow as if it were golden ducats.

From Alessio Piemontese (Ruscelli):

> To make a redde colour for the face. Take red sandal [that is sandalwood] finely stamped and strong vinegar twice distilled then put into it as much sandal as you will and let it boile faire and softely and put to it also a little rock alume stamped and you shal have a very perfect red

'Dying the eyebrows', from the *Ninth Book of Natural Magic* by John Baptiste Porta:

Take Labdanum [a brown resin obtained from the rock rose] and beat it with wine and mingle oil of myrtles with and make a very thick ointment. Or infused in oil the black leaves of the myrtle tree with a double quantity of galls bruised and use that. I use this. Galls fried in oil and they are ground with a little salt ammoniac. And mingled with vinegar wherein the pills [probably berries] of the mulberry and bramble have been boiled. With these anoint the eyebrows and let it abide all night. Then wash it off with water.

5

THE SEVENTEENTH CENTURY:
WITCHES, VIZARDS AND PATCHES

> Women are books, and men the readers be
> In whom ofte times they great Errata's see
> Here sometimes wee a blot, there we espy
> A leafe misplac'd, as least a line awry.
>
> Anon. (1640)

Introduction

Wearing cosmetics had become more popular, more acceptable and a good deal more widespread in late fifteenth and sixteenth century Europe. Building on this popularity and despite continued criticism from some quarters, in the seventeenth century a trend for wearing heavy and obvious make-up emerged. In the fashionable cities across Europe, this heavy make-up was worn not only by women but by some men too, and (in the first instance at least) especially by those women, and men, who belonged to the upper echelons of society. However, the wealthy were not alone in their taste for beauty products. As had been the case in the preceding hundred years, the middle classes copied any changes in fashion, when and where they could afford to do so. The major cities in Italy and France, in particular, were centres for the manufacture of luxury goods including cosmetics and perfumes, but there was a wide choice of beauty products (and the ingredients to make these) on the market, including cheaper alternatives to the more expensive powders and paints.

In Britain, make-up was very popular at the beginning of the seventeenth century and at its close. The prolific writer, diarist and garden enthusiast John Evelyn (1620–1706), from whom the present day cosmetic company Crabtree and Evelyn in part takes its name, remarked that in the first half of the seventeenth century, 'women began to paint themselves again, formerly a most ignominious thing and only by prostitutes'. Evelyn's observation was not, in fact very accurate as women, particularly those who belonged to the upper classes and certainly not only those working in the sex trade, had been applying cosmetics for some time. However, his comment may reflect the noticeable increase in the obvious use of make-up that was worn by many women, and men, in the seventeenth century. The poet Antony Nixon, a contemporary of Evelyn's, agreed with him regarding the sheer numbers, mostly women, wearing make-up; he remarks that 'a rare face if it not be painted' (*A Straunge Foot Post*, 1613).

Despite the popularity of cosmetics at either end of the seventeenth century in England, during the Civil Wars and the Commonwealth when the Puritans – who adhered to a strict interpretation of the scriptures – held the reins of power, fashions and styles in make-up did, for a time, become far more subdued. In the mid-seventeenth century there was even a legal attempt to restrict the extravagant and vulgar wearing of cosmetics, when the politically powerful Puritans proposed 'an act against the vice of painting and wearing black patches and immodest dresses of woman to be read[in parliament] on Friday morning next'. Though this proposed legislation did indeed receive its first reading in parliament in 1650, it got no further – and never became law. The restoration of the monarchy in 1660 not only brought the return of Charles II to the throne but also heralded a return to that lack of subtlety in terms of appearance (though not everyone adopted this) in keeping with the fashion elsewhere in Europe. French and Italian fashions spread to Britain, and the English court again became known for its style. The feel-good factor after the dourness of the Puritans and also perhaps the culture of celebrity that surrounded the rulers of some European countries, for example Queen Henrietta Maria of France, by the relevant date the widow of Charles I, to whom the recipes contained in the text *The Queens' Closet Opened* published in 1655 are attributed, may have contributed to this upsurge in women and men 'painting' themselves, as applying one's make-up was commonly referred to at this time. *The Queens Closet Opened, a* mixture of cookery and medical treatments as well as cosmetics, claims to contain 'incomparable secrets ... as they were presented to the Queen by the most experienced persons of our times'. The queen frequently took part in masques or tableaux in which she played the part of Beauty, an essential part of her real persona, which she strove to keep through the application of make-up. Indeed, the enthusiasm for wearing cosmetics prompted the poet and royalist supporter Samuel Butler (1613–1680) to compose the following pithy and consequentially memorable line as part of his satirical poem *Hudibras* (published in three parts between 1663 and 1678) 'not ten among a thousand weare their own complexion or their haire.'

Attitudes to Cosmetics

One dominant term for make-up in the seventeenth century was *fucus*. This was an old Latin word, which originally meant red dye but also referred to something that was considered gaudy or tasteless. The use of the word expresses the duality of thought that, despite its popularity, still existed as regards the buying and the wearing of make-up. While beauty products were popular and all-pervasive, at the same time they were viewed by some as tawdry and, according to contemporary rhetoric, applied by women, in the main, of low moral standards with an intention to trick or deceive. For example, Thomas Hall in his treatise entitled *The Loathsomnesse of Long Haire* (1653), states that 'this painting and disguising of faces is no better than dissimulation and lying'. Many still condemned those women who used cosmetics as immoral and considered the fact that they did so tantamount to sporting a badge of prostitution.

This continued opposition to make-up was championed, as it had been since medieval times, by the Church. The strong antipathy of religious men (and women) to cosmetics is voiced clearly in the words of Thomas Tuke, the minister at St Giles in the Fields, London: 'What a contempt of God is this, to preferre the worke of thine own finger to the worke of God'. If we take account of the literal nature of religious belief at this time, then we can say that in the following statement Tuke goes even further: 'What shall God say to such in the last judgment when they shall appear thus masked before him with these artifices' he says, 'Friends I know you not neither do I hold you for my creatures for these are not the faces that I formed'. The seventeenth-century poet Arthur Dowton expresses in just a few lines the centuries-old rhetoric, namely the unattractiveness of aging, the use of cosmetics to cover this up, and the immoral lifestyle of those who used these things:

> A loam wall and painted face are one
> for the beauty of them both is quickly gone.
> When the loam is fallen off then the lathes appear,
> so wrinkles in that face from th'eye to th'ear,
> the chastest of your sex condemn these arts,
> and many that use them have rid in carts.

In fact, loam or clay as a building material was not far removed in reality from the materials used to paint one's face at this time. Associations, both direct and indirect, with cosmetics and the building trade were long established by the seventeenth century. The Roman satirist Juvenal had not shrunk from referring to women 'plastering' their faces, a metaphor borrowed from Roman house building techniques, while others like Pliny the Elder acknowledged that the dyes that were used to tint one's hair, for example, were the same as those used to paint frescos on interior house walls. Dowton's words conjure up the same allusion. The reference to carts in his statement highlights the link between make-up and those of low moral standards – lower class prostitutes or criminals were likely to be transported to the gallows in this manner.

Some authors such as John Evelyn, and his daughter Mary, were prepared to accept some use of cosmetics but preferred the rather more reserved English style of make-up, parodying extravagant French fashion in their works entitled *The Fop's Dictionary* and *Mundus Muliebris (World of Women)*. It is, in fact, in the book *The Fop's Dictionary*, a satirical work on the language of cosmetics, that may have been written jointly by John and Mary, that the word cosmetic itself, makes an early appearance. In his text, 'cosmeticks' are defined as substances 'here used for any effeminate ornament, also artificial complexions and perfumes'.

According to Thomas Jeamson, both a physician and the author of a book entitled *Artificial Embellishments* (1665) there were a number of good reasons why women, in particular, could legitimately wear make-up and indeed should do so. To this end, he included instruction on

... how to cleanse the sweatie and sluttish complexion ... how to polish the skin when it is disfigured with scars or the marks of small pox ... to cure redness and fiery pimples in the face ... to whiten a tan'd visage and keep the face from sunburn ... how to help the complexion when it is marr'd with blue and congealed blood or black and blue proceeding from a stroak or bruise ... Remedies for the face when it is burnt or scalded... to beautye the face howsoever disfigured.

The justifiable reasons Jeamson gives for applying make-up centre around the effects of disease and disfigurement, that is, cosmetics used to remedy accident or misfortune.

Other writing on the subject promoted beauty products too, believing their use was a wife's duty to her husband and that by making the best of herself a woman might please her husband accordingly. The English poet and writer Richard Braithwaite, (1588–1673) in his book *The English Gentlewoman,* first published in 1631, argued for women to be allowed to use cosmetics without judgement for this reason. 'In some cases women might use their painting and powdering without sin; first if it were to the intent to cover any blemishes or deformity; secondly if the husband commanded it'. His statement brings to mind the degree of authority that the husband at this time might exercise in relation to his wife in this as in other matters. However, others held contrasting opinions. A work entitled *The Ladies Dictionary* published in 1694 subtitled as '*an entertainment for women*' stated that 'A painted face is enough to destroy the reputation of her who uses it'. It seems that the author wanted women to enjoy reading about make-up but to refrain from using too much of it themselves.

Nature and Artifice

It is certainly true to say there was great strength of feeling on both sides of the argument as to whether to wear or not to wear make-up. The deeper and more philosophical aspects of these arguments revolved around which was superior – nature or artifice. This too was a debate that had existed in the past and would continue to be a matter of concern and discussion far beyond the seventeenth century. According to John Bulwer, the

English novelist and statesman, 'our English ladies ... seeme to have borrowed some of their cosmetical from Barbarous nations; too much paint recalled the origins of make-up in the body paint of primitive man.' Aristocratic fashionable ladies of the time would hardly have appreciated the comparison. Rhetorically speaking, it seems women in particular were damned if they did apply cosmetics and damned if they did not. In reality, however, there was some middle ground. For example, skin care products and tooth cleaners were not frowned upon to the same extent as rouge or hair dye, which sought to alter the natural appearance rather than simply to maintain it. Also despite a trend among many for quite obvious powder and paint, there was also an appreciation of the art of applying make-up that was both subtle and effective. Regardless of differences of opinion, however, by the second half of the seventeenth century, make-up, to a greater or lesser extent, was *de rigueur*, especially among women. The long association with women of loose morals or those in the sex trade (the prostitute had become a virtual metaphor for make-up) had always been, in reality, a fallacy. By the sixteenth century, as I have noted, even royalty had their names associated with cosmetics manuals. The trend continued in the seventeenth century.

Men indulged in the use of beauty products too, especially for the purposes of maintaining their hair (whether their own or a wig) and their beards (when they were in fashion) as well as to clear their skin and to prevent body odour. Even the most famous Puritan of them all, Oliver Cromwell, Lord Protector (1653–58), owned and most probably used make-up in some form or other. Despite this widespread use, there is plenty of anti-cosmetic sentiment to be found in poetry, prose and plays. In stereotypical fashion and in a plain style that reinforces his preference, the poet Alexander Brome (1620–1666) comes out on the side of nature in his poem, *To a Painted Lady*:

leave these deluding tricks and shows
be honest and downright
what nature did to view expose
do you keep out of sight
The novice youth may chance admire
your dressing paints and spells ...
you need no pains or time to waste
to set your beauties forth
with oyles and paint and drugs and cost
more than the face is worth
Nature herself her own work does
and hates all needless arts.

Writing about Cosmetics

Household books continued to find popularity. These were especially prolific in the second half of the seventeenth century, mixing recipes for cosmetics with cookery, prescriptions for medical remedies and advice about cleaning agents. Many, like Gervase Markham (1568–1637) whose *Book of Housewifery* was first published in 1615, ran to a second edition or more. Although this may seem a bit of a farrago in terms of content to us, none would have questioned the topics contained within the pages of these manuals at the time. As Markham puts it, her book contains 'the inward and outward which ought to be in a complete woman. As her skill in physics, cookery, banqueting stuff, distillation, perfumes, wool, hemp, flax, dairies, brewing, baking and all other things belonging to a household'. Some of the topics covered, particularly medicines and make-up, had a long history in terms of association, while all encompassed knowledge considered the responsibility of the women of the household. In addition, the skill involved in the preparation of a cosmetic product in the home was very similar, if not identical, to the expertise required in the preparation of food – methods such as heating, mixing, pounding, grinding, making a decoction (boiling down or reducing), straining and distilling were used in cooking and also in the making of cosmetics. Whether a woman, as mistress of the house, oversaw these procedures or whether as a servant, she actually carried out these multifarious tasks, a woman's work in the seventeenth century, it seems, was never done.

A new source of information as regards cosmetics and their application aimed at avid women readers first began to emerge in the seventeenth century. *The Ladies Mercury*, an offshoot from *The Athenian Mercury*, a periodical with a readership of both sexes lasted only four weeks but marked the beginning of what would become a burgeoning market in women's magazines. *The Ladies Mercury* took the form of a single sheet printed on both sides covering a range of matters thought to be of interest to a female readership, including advice on the wearing of make-up and advertisements for cosmetic products. However, we must wait until the following century for the prolific output in magazines that would be influential both in terms of what, as well as how, women wore make-up.

Trade

With the founding of The East India Company in 1601, trade in luxury goods, which included cosmetics and perfumes, flourished. Bears' grease applied as a skin care treatment was imported into Europe from Russia and Canada. Soap and perfumed ointments came from Aleppo in the Levant. Pharmacies sold the raw materials with which to make a cosmetic. Aside from these shop outlets, iterant street sellers could be found selling beauty products – especially in the larger towns and cities. Supply would not always have met demand and this may explain why some recipes for powders and paints were made up at home in bulk as people took advantage of the ingredients when they were available. Women, including those who belonged to the better classes, who were down on their luck might turn to selling beauty products as a means of earning a living. In one of her plays, Margaret Cavendish (1623–73) both aristocrat (she was the Duchess of Newcastle upon Tyne) and writer, includes just such a character called Lady Poverty who, because she is in matrimonial trouble, turns to making and selling cosmetics in order to support herself financially. Dorothea Dury, the wife of the Scottish Calvinist minister and educational reformer John Dury (1596–1680), (she herself was active in the field especially of education for women), may be one real life example.

Those who were in the business of selling cosmetics naturally had a vested interest in justifying as well as promoting the use of their beauty products. Dr Stephen Draper, a businessman, commented 'Ladies, beauty is a blessing from God, and everyone ought to preserve it ... they do as much offend that neglect it as they do that paint their faces'. Thomas Platters the Younger (1574–1628), a Swiss physician and seasoned traveller, recalling his adventures in England noted that 'lotions potions ointments and creames were churned out by alchemical confidence tricksters or in the still rooms and bed chambers of country houses'. The lady (or gentleman) needed to acquire her cosmetics from a reliable source.

Health and Hygiene

The English naturalist and writer John Ray (1625–1705) included the following in his handbook of proverbs produced in 1670: 'Wash your hands often, your feet seldom and your head never'. Hand washing certainly minimised the spread of germs and was widely practised even though contemporary society did not fully understand how infections were contracted. While the infrequent cleansing of other parts of the body is of course alien to the modern concept of hygiene, the ideas expressed in this pithy proverb are perfectly rational within their contemporary historical context.

There was, after all, a real danger of death if one caught so much as a cold in the seventeenth century.

Washing of the head at this time referred to washing one's hair. The diarist John Evelyn tells us that he washed his hair just once a year using warm water and sweet herbs to do so. While he claimed to find the experience pleasant, Evelyn also believed that the effect of this annual ritual would keep his hair clean for the rest of the year and seems to have been in no hurry to carry out the process more regularly, perhaps for fear of catching a cold or a fever.

The Beautiful Woman

Margaret Cavendish, the said Duchess of Newcastle upon Tyne, summarised the essential components of female beauty in her poem *Dialogue betwixt Wit and Beauty* in the following lines; 'Body perfect made Complexion pure,' hair that is 'thick, and long, curl'd to the feet'. In his poem *A Celebration of Charis*, one of the Three Graces in Greek mythology, the poet and playwright Ben Jonson (1572–1637), goes into a little more detail. He describes the eponymous woman (that is Charis) as a maiden with 'a complexion of milke and roses', 'a smooth forehead', 'a white and polished neck,' 'sparkling eyes', 'cherry lips', 'arched eyebrows' and 'bright golden hair'. In terms of the standard of beauty, it appears nothing much had changed since the days of Greece and Rome; the pale complexion, large eyes and just a hint of colour are still very much in vogue. However, the means of achieving such perfection was not only subject to the ebb and flow of fashion but also altered by means of the arrival of new ideas, methods and the availability of new materials with which to effect such an appearance.

Youth and Beauty

The story of the ancient Greek prostitute Phryne was a favourite myth and morality tale among seventeenth century writers.

According to legend, Phryne was playing a game of Follow my Leader and, when it came to her turn to choose, she chose water with which she duly washed her face. When the others in the game copied her all their make-up came off and they were shown to be, in truth, old hags. Phyrne, on the other hand, was young and beautiful and wore no make-up and therefore looked just as lovely once she had washed her face. The moral of the tale is of course that youth, as ever, was an essential element of beauty and to beware of old women who were among the most likely to try to hide their true appearance behind a mask of make-up. In John Marston's play, *The Malcontent,* one of the characters Maquerelle, a rather aged lady-in-waiting says 'but when our beauty fades goodnight with us. There cannot be an uglier thing to see than an old woman from which a pruning pinching painting deliver all sweet beauties'. The sentiments conveyed here are no different to those expressed by the Roman satirist Juvenal. The cruel rhyming couplet penned by Sir George Etherege (1635–1692) in his comedy of manners entitled *The Man of Mode* is equally harsh but not completely devoid of reality at this time. He remarks that a woman is 'Past her prime at twenty, decayed at four and twenty and old and insufferable at thirty'. Women relied on their looks for social and financial security and growing old might not be something done willingly or indeed gracefully.

Men and Make-up

Thomas Hall in his treatise *The Loathsomeness of Long Hair* asserts that, 'a decent growth of the beard is a signe of manhood ... given by God to distinguish the male from the female sex'. Men certainly used beauty products to care for any facial hair. Jeamson includes a recipe for dyeing the beard 'black as jet' using a mixture of walnut shells, oak roots and good quality red wine strained and mixed with myrtle and stirred together having been left out to sit in the sun. The heavy bottomed wigs they wore were also an expression of both masculinity and of great wealth. The English writer James Cleland, author of *The Institution of a Young Nobleman* (1607), writes, with reference to young noblemen, 'some cannot be content as God made them but as though they were bundled up in haste and sent into the world not fully finished must use drugs, balms, ointments paintings lac virginale and what not?' There is evidence of a burgeoning interest in make-up for men that would grow stronger in the following century. In the seventeenth century, however, individual men, some in prominent positions or even at the very pinnacle of their careers in public life, certainly did take to wearing aids to beauty. James II employed herbalist George Wilson who prescribed for the king a face lotion made of lemon rind, coriander, vanilla pods, cloves, nutmegs, storax (a sweet gum resin), benzoin gum (another resin still used as a preservative and skin restorer in modern make-up) and lastly honey. While the legal fraternity wore wigs as part of their dress in court, Judge Jeffreys, Chief Justice of the King's Bench and Lord Chancellor, and known more colloquially as the hanging judge, not only sported the obligatory wig but sentenced those brought before him harshly while wearing heavy make-up.

The Tools of the Toilette

Mirrors, combs and other implements pertaining to the toilette became more portable and therefore more adaptable in the seventeenth century. For example, a lady or gentleman might carry a small pocket mirror, known as a sprunking mirror, that allowed the owner to check easily and discreetly that his or her make-up was up to scratch. These were expensive and much-valued possessions with decorative frames made of silver, ivory or carved wood. Boxes, bottles, jars, and other containers for cosmetics might be on public display in the receiving rooms where the rich and famous greeted their guests, sometimes when they were in the process of getting dressed. Elaborate cosmetic pots made of fine silver, glass or fine china on public display might also be laid out to impress potential suitors of the daughter or daughters of the house. The objects themselves, as well as their contents, conveyed a message of the wealth and importance of the owner to those who came to visit and conduct business in their houses.

Hannah Woolley

Hannah Woolley (1622–75) originally worked as a servant girl, possibly to Lady Anne Maynard a member of the British aristocracy who sat for the famous portrait painter Thomas Gainsborough. Upon Hannah's fortuitous and happy marriage to schoolmaster Jerome Woolley, she opened a school with him but also found time to expand her interest in all things medicinal and cosmetic, basing her recipes on the knowledge that she had inherited from her mother and sisters. On the death of her husband in 1661, although she did briefly remarry, Hannah turned, by and large, to publishing the knowledge she had acquired in a number of books on household management. She appears to have written both to further her own interests and also to support herself financially. Although she had to finance her first book entitled *The Ladies Directory* herself in 1661 her work proved popular, and not only was this title reprinted a few years later, it was followed by a number of other books. In Hannah's *Accomplished Ladies Delight* (1670) the intended audience is the mistress of the house herself. The author is at pains to explain exactly what her book will cover and there are a number of products whose use is attributed to, and therefore tacitly endorsed, by individual women of note even if we are not entirely sure who they were: for example, 'an excellent beauty water used by the D of C'. In her book *The Gentlewoman's Companion*, first printed in 1675, Hannah Woolley included recipes or receipts 'to correct a stinking breath' and 'to clean the skin of your face and make it look beautiful and fair' as well a recipe for stewed oysters, how to marinate mullet and advice on how 'to stop the bleeding of a wound'. The content of such household books remained as varied as ever. Hannah Woolley's manual for working women was not published until 1677, two years after her death. The work had the lengthy title of The *Compleat Servant Maid; Or, the young maidens tutor Directing them how they may fit, and qualifie themselves for any of these employments. viz. Waiting woman, housekeeper, chambermaid, cook, maid, undercook maid, nurserymaid, dairymaid, laundrymaid, housemaid, scullery maid Composed for the great benefit and advantage of all young maidens.* Women working in the homes of the wealthy at all levels from the very lowest servant needed to have these skills, which included the preparation and application of cosmetics in order to effectively serve the lady of the house. As ever Hannah's recipes in this volume were typically varied, covering medicines, cookery and cleaning methods as well as cosmetics. When it came to make-up, many of her recipes were also specifically targeted for use to remedy a particular problem; there are individual recipes for the removal of freckles, redness and smallpox marks. In the main, Hannah used natural plant-based materials in her recipes. However, she was not opposed to using some of the dangerous ingredients such as lye, brimstone (now referred to as sulphur) and arsenic. Occasionally she gives us quantities as in the following example 'to make the face look youthful':

Take two ounces of *aqua vitae*, bean flower water and rose water each four ounces water –lilies six ounces mix them all and add to them one dram (an apothecaries' measure) of the whitest tragacanth, set it I the sun six days then strain it through a fine linen cloth wash your face with it in the morning and do not wipe it off.

This pleasant-sounding mixture, given the quality and cost of ingredients, was one for the use of the very wealthy only.

Skin Care

Good skin has always been an asset. In the seventeenth century an unblemished complexion was not only recognised as one element of great beauty, but was also deemed a good indication that she, or he, was free from some of the more noxious contagious diseases of the time, chiefly syphilis or smallpox. While Oliver Cromwell famously may have wanted to have his portrait painted 'warts and all', there is concrete evidence that even he did not neglect the care for his appearance entirely. The Cromwell Museum in Huntingdon has in its possession a chest given to Cromwell as a gift from The Duke of Tuscany. This fine wooden container housed in all fifty-five pots of ointments. When these ointments were analysed they were found to be expensively perfumed with jasmine, cassia and orange blossom. Cromwell's soap was made with olive oil. As there is little left in any of these containers, it seems logical to suggest that Cromwell himself may have enjoyed using these scented mixtures to care for his skin.

Mercury and lead continued to be popular as skin care remedies although there was no shortage of contemporary comment on just how much harm could be done by applying such cosmetics. Doctor Fierovant, a seventeenth-century physician, warns those who might be tempted to use sublimate of mercury that it is

...malignant, and biting [and] corrosive: if it bee put upon mans flesh it burneth it in a short space, mortifying the place, not without great paine to the patient. Wherefore such women as vase it about their face, hue always black teeth, standing far out of their gums like a Spanish mule; an offensive breath, with a face halfe scorched, and an unclean complexion. So that simple women thinking to grow more beautiful, become disfigured, hastening olde age before the time, and giving occasion to their husbandes to seeke strangers instead of their wiues; with divers other inconveniences.

Ceruse or white lead was eventually classified as a poison in 1634, this only after centuries of use as a cosmetic – and it didn't stop there. Even the legal recognition of the dangers of applying this did not put people off. White lead would continue to be used not only for years but for centuries to come.

An anonymous text from 1608 entitled *The Closet for Ladies and Gentlewomen* recommends the application of what sounds similar to a full English breakfast upon one's face: 'Take fresh bacon grease and the whites of eggs' the recipe says, 'and stamp them together and a little powder of bays and anoint your face therewith and it will make it white'. Certainly grease is a very basic moisturiser. In addition, the application of the white part of the egg is possibly an example of the belief in sympathetic magic where the colour of the egg could be transferred to the face given that only the white should be used. Eggs do, however, contain vitamins that can be beneficial to the skin and continue to be used in modern cosmetics for this reason. One seventeenth century herbal recommends lemon juice mixed with salt or brimstone, oil of turpentine and fresh cream to eliminate spots. Bismuth, a white metallic substance derived from nickel, tin or silver, at this time a treatment for syphilis, was also used as a foundation though some might find that it had the opposite effect and aggravated the skin. Pearl powder made from pearls dissolved in an acid, either vinegar or lemon juice, were ground to a powder and applied to produce an even skin tone. A prized and expensive product, pearl powder was only an option for those who had money to spend. Burnt animal bones, of pig for example, mixed with poppy oil for easy application or rice powder were cheaper alternatives. Sir Hugh Plat included the following recipe as a cure for a 'face that is red or pimpled', 'Dissolve common salt in the juice of lemons and with a linen cloth pat the patient's face that is full of heat or pimples. It cures in a few dressings.' Women were often criticised because of the thickness of the make-up they might wear to cover up the extensive damage done to the skin either by disease or indeed by the dangerous cosmetics that they had applied in the first place. Thomas Tuke asserts, 'A man might easily cut off a curd or cheesecake from either of [women's] cheekes'.

Cosmetics and Witchcraft

A lovely face has a great power to attract men's souls and inflame their bodies.

Moderata Fonte, The *Worth of Women*, 1600

No one doubts the power of great beauty. However it was not only the prostitute, painted like a sign advertising her business, or the scheming mistress, her heart set on a good marriage, that might use their looks to secure a man. In the seventeenth century, when accusations of witchcraft were at their height, women who had the ability by means of their great beauty to seduce men, as well as women known to produce or sell cosmetic products whether in innocence or where these might be construed as a cover for more harmful purposes, laid themselves open to accusations of witchcraft.

Particular blemishes and even certain physical features could be interpreted as an indication of sorcery. Freckles, for example, are not something the modern woman would concern herself with, but getting rid of freckles for those living in the seventeenth century, particularly for women, was very important as these blemishes could be considered the marks of evil. Suffice to say if we consider freckles in the context of the accusations of witchcraft and ensuing witch hunts that took place in the seventeenth century, then these marks become a very serious matter indeed. Some of the recipes that purported to eliminate freckles do sound like something akin to magic themselves, not so much with regard to their ingredients but because of the language and other components of the recipes. One remedy of long standing, in use since Roman times, consisted of a bread poultice left on overnight and washed off in the morning with a mixture of bran and water or violet water. Sap from the birch tree was also reputed to get rid of freckles. The sheer number of different recipes aimed at removing them is testament to the level of concern there was about these marks at this time, also to the difficulty, if not impossibility, of getting rid of them if you had them in the first place, and to the serious consequences when these were cited as proof someone was a witch. A pamphlet written by minister Thomas Tuke and published in 1616 places cosmetics and witchcraft firmly together by including both in the title of his work, *A discourse against painting and tincturing of women: wherein the abominable sinnes of murther and poisoning pride and ambition adultery and witchcraft are set forth and discourse, whereunto is added the picture of a picture or the character of a painted woman*; a long title for a short work. Other works made the same connection and the preference for long convoluted titles made making the link, or at least the suggestion of it, simple from the very start. For example in *Wonder of Wonders or a Metamorphosis of Fair Faces Voluntarily Transformed into Foul Visages or an invective against black spotted faces* written by an unidentified author under the pseudonym of *Miso Spilus* (Latin for 'I hate spots') published in 1662 states,

> Phantastic madams that are not content
> with god's design but think to ronamanet
> youselves with borrowed foils of patch and paint
> whereby you shew more of the witch than saint.

Rouge

The importance of blushing for women and indeed the importance of being seen to blush at the right moment cannot be underestimated. In the words of Thomas Tuke in his discourse *Against Painting and Tincturing of Women*; 'It is not good enough to be good but she that is good must seem good; she that is chaste must seem chaste; she that is humble must seem humble; she that is modest must seem to be so and not plaster her face so she cannot blush'. Those who objected to make-up *per se* often commented on blusher being applied too thickly by the wearer. As a man of the Church, Tuke expresses the accepted view of cosmetics within the context of his religious beliefs; that is, as a sin against God and a futile and corrupt attempt to improve upon nature. However, a demure and well-timed blush was not just something revered by those belonging to the Church hierarchy but had appeared as an important element of the delicate feminine, pure and morally upright woman in much earlier classical poetry. However, a natural blush is difficult to feign as it is an instinctive reaction induced by emotion that cannot be easily controlled. The aim of rouge was to produce a natural blush but one that could be controlled by the wearer as it was false rather than a natural response and there were those as far back in time as the early Roman Empire (the poet Ovid for example) who understood the benefits of being able to manage a blush by having it painted on. One of Thomas Jeamson's many recipes in *Artificial embellishments or Arts best directions how to preserve beauty or procure it.* (1665) reads as follows:

Take madder, frankincense, myrrhe, oriental saffron, mastick, of each like quantities, bruise them all, and steep them in white wine, anoint the face therewith going to bed, in the morning wash either with cold or warm water, it will purple any part with a gallant and pleasing blush.

Or, 'Take fraxinella roots (an aromatic plant with white flowers), chew them, and tye them in a fine ragg, and bathe the face.' Jeamson's latter suggestion was a much cheaper option. His first recipe in particular is packed with expensive ingredients. Vermillion and cinnabar were both toxic but worn as blusher, despite the known dangers. Safer alternatives including dragon's blood, a harmless resin, cochineal, alkanet, brazilwood and even red iron oxide or rust, were also applied as rouge. Red ochre, around since prehistoric times, was still worn by the poorer classes. Spanish wool, paper or leather, basically materials imbued with red dye, were all means of adding a little colour to one's complexion. As well as applying rouge, older women sometimes resorted to cheek plumpers to fill out their cheeks, sunken with age, and thus improve their appearance. John Evelyn described plumpers as 'certain very thin round and light balls to plump out and fill up the cavities of the cheeks much us'd by old court-countesses'. These were, in fact, herb-filled pomander balls, which apart from filling out the cheeks and maybe even drawing attention to one's rouge at the same time, must have made it difficult to speak. Suffice to say, fake or genuine, the interpretation of the blush as an expression of a woman's moral character and therefore social worth was one that was widely understood and again underlines the importance of getting one's appearance just right.

Hands

The juice from the common plant sorrel could be applied to one's hands to make them appear white. This would certainly have been a cheap option as sorrel grew, and still does grow, wild in abundance along hedgerows and country lanes or on almost any patch of waste ground. Sorrel may have been more easily accessed by those living in the countryside perhaps than for the population in the towns and cities. Hands that were rough were an indication that their owner was engaged in manual labour and therefore someone of low social status. Christopher Wirsung in his work *General Practise of Physicke* (1654), 'for all persons whatsoever' includes the following remedy for chapped hands using a selection of ingredients that would have been easily found in the well-stocked kitchen in the home of a wealthy family:

Melt three ounces of fresh butter and three ounces of suet of hart [deer] and cut four or five apples into it; add six ounces of white wine and boil until the apples are soft; add half a dram of cinnamon, camphor, cloves and nutmeg, two ounces of rosewater and boil this until the rosewater has evaporated; finally strain through a cloth.

Some attention was paid to the nails, at least to encourage their growth and maintain their condition, if not in the sense of applying colour. According to Hannah Woolley, to make the nails grow 'take wheat flower and mingle it with honey and lay it to the nails and it will help them'. Thomas Jeamson employs the well-worn epithet of roses and lilies to describe a lady's hands and advises 'to adde the roses sweetness to the lillied loveliness of your snow hands scent your gloves'. Gloves were not only worn as protection but when scented of course imparted their pleasant odour and no doubt on occasion concealed unsightly hands.

Hair

In general, instead of washing their hair, men and women kept their hair clean by combing it frequently. Care of the hair was an essential part of daily personal grooming. There was, however, some incentive to wash one's hair on a more regular basis as Gervase Markham points out; 'rosemary water (the face washed therein both morning and night) causeth a fair and clear countenance. Also the head washed therewith and let dry of itself preserveth the falling of the hair and causeth more to grow'. For men, as well as women, a full head of hair was an indication of good health. In the seventeenth century the length of a man's hair could even denote his political allegiance. The royalist Cavaliers wore their hair long, while the Parliamentarians or Roundheads had their hair cropped short. There was little chance of getting the two confused. Women did not cut their hair. Instead, various remedies purported to make hair grow thick and strong. The following recipe 'to grow thicken and curl the hair' comes from a cookbook called *The Queens's Delight* and subtitled *The Art of Preserving, Conserving and Candying. and also, A right Knowledge of making Perfumes, and Distilling the most Excellent Waters;*

> Take half a pound of Aqua Mellis in the Spring time of the year, warm a little of it every Morning when you rise in a Sawcer, and tie a little spunge to a fine box comb, and dip it in the water, and therewith moisten the roots of the Hair in combing it, and it will grow long, thick, and curled in a very short time.

To thicken hair Hannah Woolley suggested lye soap (caustic soda) mixed with the ashes of burnt frogs or goat dung. The smell would hardly endear such a product to its user today and the caustic soda then and now was likely to do more harm than good. The French chemist Nicholas Lemery (1645–1715) proposed 'Wash[ing] in your own urine or with rosewater mixed with wine else make a decoction of the rinds of lemon'. We do know that women, at least, used lead combs to blacken their eyebrows. *The Ladies Dictionary* also recommends a mixture of hazelnuts and goats' grease to make eyebrows 'a very curious black'. While there is some suggestion that eye make-up was worn, Bulwer criticises women for 'drawing circles around their eyes'. A little shading above the eyes in portrait may indicate the presence of eye shadow though this may equally simply be artistic licence.

In the first half of the seventeenth century beards, which required some care and attention, were popular and considered and a sign of manhood and maturity. However by the middle of the century, fashions had changed and the clean-shaven look was back in vogue. The diarist Samuel Pepys used pumice stone to remove the hair from his face as he found this 'very easy and cleanly'. A visit to the barbers might involve the use of a razor to shave off one's beard. This required the labour-intensive task of fetching of hot water. Barbers worked hard at all times of the day in their own shops, though sometimes such establishments did acquire the reputation for being little more than gossip shops or drinking dens. Barber's shops were not exclusively for the use of men. Women, though not the most respectable in society, might also have their hair arranged or dressed there. Barbers might also visit the homes of wealthy clients, on request.

According to *The Ladies Dictionary* (1694) 'as for the colour of the hair, opinions are various ... but above all it should not be red'. It seems some things had changed since the days of Elizabeth I, whose red hair was one of her most distinctive and admired features. In the seventeenth century red hair, which had been associated with slaves in the classical world but gained some popularity in the Middle Ages to become briefly fashionable under Queen Elizabeth, now assumed a connection with witchcraft. This association possibly arose from the fact that naturally red hair is relatively rare and those who have red hair often possess other more unusual features such as green eyes as well as freckles, known in the seventeenth century as marks of the devil. Natural plant dyes like the expensive saffron were still available for those who wanted blonde hair and could afford the price. However there was quite a fashion for brunettes. One recipe for a chestnut brown hair dye suggests applying a highly dangerous mixture of lead, sulphur and quick lime thinned with water and leaving this mixture on for fifteen minutes before rinsing it off.

Pomades were mostly made from bear fat so a pleasantly scented hair powder (these were generally based on a starch made from rice or other cereal plants) might be an effective way of disguising the less attractive odour of animal fat and sopping up any excess grease. Thomas Jeamson in his work *Artificial Embellishments* is not being facetious with reference to hair powders when he says:

If after you have used all hitherto commended pomanders ye meet with any that defies your charms and is obstinate do not yet despair ladies for this chapter teaches ye how ye shall tickle his nose and fetch him about with a powder which will give ye so rich a scent that the rose and violets in all your cheeks shall not make ye half so sweet.

He goes on to describe a mixture of orris root, cloves, and storax mixed with starch or rice powder to be applied to the hair. Women expected great things from their cosmetics, including snaring a husband. Hair powders were worn by both men and women and were intended to attract the opposite sex by means of their pleasant smell. However, they would also have helped to keep one's hair style in place and reduce the need for washing. The scent of roses was a popular fragrance. Simon Barbe in his book *The French Perfumer* (1696) offers the following recipe:

Put a Pound of Rose leaves to twenty Pounds of Starch powder in a Box, mix them all together with your hand very well, and every four hours shake them well, that the flowers should not heat; the next day at the same time you put them in the Box, sift them and put as many roses again, and so for three times; all that while you must let the box be open, from the first time you put the flowers in, till you take them out, and your powder will be made.

Wigs

Louis XIV, King of France, suffered from hair loss from the age of seventeen and was at pains to conceal this fact. To this end the king employed numerous wigmakers. The image he projected became a trend that the court, upper and middle classes were quick to follow. Full powdered wigs, in particular, became increasingly popular. The cost of a wig was considerable, especially if it were an elaborate one, so the wearing of a wig became a means of signalling one's wealth and importance and, as wigs were of value, wig snatching became a common crime. Women tended to build on their own hair with hair-pieces and other extras, rather than wear a full wig. The best wigs were made from human hair. Wigs were not without their problems, even when carrying out ordinary daily tasks. Samuel Pepys' entry in his diary for 28 September 1668 says, 'here also standing by a candle that was brought in for sealing a letter so set my periwig a fire which made such an odd noise. Nobody could tell what it was till they saw the flame, my back being to the candle'. Despite the potential for mishaps, wigs were popular and men instead of hiding the fact they wore them often drew attention to that fact and even combed their wigs in public as a sort of leisure activity. There were advantages too. Wearing a wig did to some extent mitigate the perennial problem of head lice. Although nits were as attracted to a wig as they were to a natural head of hair it was much easier to send an infested wig to be deloused (by boiling) than it was to rid one's own hair of such an infestation, and subsequently keep this at bay.

Hair Removal

The Queen's Closet Opened offers alternatives for the removal of unwanted hair. 'Take the shells of fifty two eggs beat them small and distil them with a god fire and with the water anoint yourself where you would have the hair off'. Or else 'cat's dung that is hard and dried beaten to powder and tempered with strong vinegar and anointed to the place'. Vigorous preparation is required for both. A large supply of eggs are needed for the first recipe while the latter would certainly have had a strong smell. At least neither could be described as dangerous. The forehead is not an area that we would think of removing hair from but in the seventeenth century, as had been the case in the Middle Ages, a high forehead was considered desirable in a woman. To quote Thomas Jeamson 'The forehead is the ivory throne where beauty sits in state.' His accolade clearly indicates that a high forehead was a much-admired feature. He goes on explain the means of attaining this look; 'to make the forehead high eradicate the hairs which encroach too much. Take as much mastick as you shall have occasion to use and steep it in warm water till it be so soft that you can spread it.' This was tied down and washed off in the morning. No doubt the sticky substance, effectively a glue, took the offending strands of hair with it when peeled off. Jeamson also recommends 'to keep the hair from growing again there is quicklime and henbane mixed with arsenic'; hardly a safe means of hair removal.

Lips and Teeth

The fashion as far as women were concerned was for small mouths painted with the same substances that might be applied as rouge. All lipstick came in some shade of red. For chapped lips 'Rub them with the sweat behind your ears and this will make them smooth and well coloured', says Hannah Woolley. While this sounds unpleasant, it is at least a remedy that requires no vast expenditure on a lot of ingredients so would be available to the poorer in society, assuming they had somehow learnt of this idea. It was important too to keep one's teeth in good order. In the early part of the century Gervase Markham in her book *The English Housewife* (1615) recommends the following for removing yellow stains from one's teeth, 'take sage and salt of each alike and stamp them well together. Then bake till it be hard and make a fine powder. Then therewith rub the teeth evening and morning and it will take away all yellowness.' The mixture itself with its abrasive qualities would have helped clean and indeed dampen down infection, though too much of this was likely to remove enamel too. Cleaning the teeth with soot, which is, of course, black seems odd but was one method employed to do exactly that in the seventeenth century.

We get the first mention of a toothbrush in 1651. Advertisements appeared marketing dentifrices. One such advertisement from 1660 reads, 'Most excellent and approved dentifrices to scour and cleanse the teeth making them white as ivory preserves from tooth ache'. This promises the earth but does not divulge its ingredients. Suffice to say it can only be purchased from 'Thomas Rookes, Stationer'. In conclusion the advert states that 'the reader is desired to beware of counterfeits'. According to Hannah Woolley, to whiten teeth one must 'take of harts-horn and horses' teeth of each 2 ounces, sea shells, coom salt, cypress nuts each 1 ounce burn them together in an oven and make a powder and work it up with the mucilage of gum tragacanth and rub the teeth there with'. In the seventeenth century it was discovered hippo ivory was a good match for human teeth though it is hard to imagine that too many hippos were readily available for this purpose.

Vizards and Patches

The vizard was a mask worn exclusively by women. This covered the whole of her face and was made from velvet with a button attached, which the wearer would hold between her teeth to keep the mask in place. Undoubtedly, the vizard added an air of mystery or feminine mystique. Think of the masqued ball. Who is the gentleman dancing with? What does the lady look like underneath her vizard? However, women didn't just wear these masks at balls but were seen out and about in public places, such as the theatre, wearing them too. Samuel Pepys in his diaries makes the following observation; 'Lady Mary Cromwell who looks as well as I have known her and well clad but when the house began to fill she put on her vizard and so kept it on all the play which of late is become a great fashion among the ladies which hides the whole face'. For a lady wearing a vizard was in fact a very practical measure. The mask not only concealed any faults from onlookers but also prevented one's make-up from smudging and protected the complexion from the elements of wind, rain and even extreme heat, which could respectively wash off or dry up a lady's make-up.

The trend for wearing face patches re-emerged first in France at the French court and then spread across the rest of Europe, copied by the lower classes, in particular those in the sex trade. In Roman times, slaves, on becoming freedmen, often wore patches made from leather softened with alum to cover up slave marks; similarly, at least to start with in the seventeenth century, these patches were seen as an effective, as well as attractive, way of concealing marks – this time caused by disease, more especially deep-seated blemishes left by smallpox. Even though it is certain that initially the placement of these patches was driven by whatever smallpox marks, spots or other blemishes one wished to conceal, once the fashion for wearing these became established some sort of code appears to have developed and the placement of these patches could indicate the status of the wearer, perhaps whether they were married or not – or even her, or his, political allegiance. Made from silk or cut from velvet, patches came in many shapes and sizes including crescent moons and stars, hearts and diamonds. The following seventeenth century street peddler's cry gives us a sense of what might be available for purchase:

Here patches are of ev'ry cut for pimples and for scars,
Here's all the wandering planet signs, and some of the fixed stars,
Already gummed to make them stick,
They need no other sky,
Nor stars for Lilly for to view to tell your fortunes by.
Come lads and lasses, what so you lack,
Here's weare if all prices
Here's long and short,
Here's wide and straight,
Here are things of all sizes.

Some contemporary writers in their eagerness to condemn the practice, saw in this fashion an association with superstition, astrology and an attempt to read the heavens. Although black patches could set off a fair complexion, sometimes too many were worn at once. The fashion would become overdone to such an extent that it was bound to draw criticism. In his *Anthropometamorphosis,* an ambitious work of an anthropological nature describing different cultures and social practices, first published in 1650, physician and author John Bulwer (c 1606–1656) makes this clear. He says that 'ladies fill their visages full of them varied into all manner of shapes.' Samuel Pepys the diarist, who was himself quick to adopt the fashion of wearing a wig, was not so quick to allow his wife to sport the latest fashion in patches though, as this entry in his diary testifies, he did relent. He remarks: 'My wife seemed very pretty today, it being the first time I had given her leave to wear a black patch.'

Cosmetics on Stage

Plays and other theatrical spectacles began to be performed indoors rather than out in the open air. This meant that those involved had to consider the impact of the light on the appearance of the actors on the stage. Make-up might also be used to accentuate facial expressions, to create a female appearance as men took the female parts in any play, or as props and to provide a theme for that ever-popular dramatic convention, the face painting scene. The playwright Ben Jonson expressed the view that 'man is read in his face'. His interest in appearance and the contrivance of appearance is marked by the number of face painting scenes in his plays. In fact there are no less than fifty references to make-up in Ben Jonson's play *The Devil is an Ass.* According to John Marston in his play *The Malcontent* (c 1603) 'But when our beauty fades, goodnight with us. There cannot be an uglier thing to see than an old woman. From which no pruning, pinching painting deliver all sweet beauties'. The theatre played on the age-old theme and genuine concern of many women in real life, that is, growing old and the loss of beauty and youth. Painted ladies, beauticians, pimps and prostitutes were as much stock characters on the early modern stage as they had been in Greek and Roman comedy. In Jonson's play *Volpone* or *The Wolf,* two of these stereotypical female characters appear, namely the innocent maiden Celia and the bawd Madam Would-Be. A quack attempts to seduce Celia with the offer of a priceless face powder while the Madame plays an important role in this staged dramatic convention, where she complains to her maids and extols the value of cosmetics in a similar vein to the much earlier example in Plautus' comedy the *Mostellaria* or *Haunted House.* Of course much of the action is satirical and therefore more of a send-up than an accurate portrayal of real life. However we can try not only to understand the joke but also to draw out what we can in the way of factual information from these references to make-up that appear quite frequently in contemporary theatre.

There is a suggestion of something akin to a backlash against the artifice of make-up reflected in the drama of the day. Sir Hugh Plat is scorned by Jonson for encouraging women to wear make-up and the dangers and disreputable associations attributed to cosmetics in real life are represented by the common theme of poisoning by cosmetics in contemporary drama. In Barnabe Barnes' *The Devil's Charter,* written and first performed in 1607, Lucrezia Borgia is poisoned by her make-up which stings and burns her cheeks and is symbolic of her own inner immorality.

The Wickedness of Cosmetics

In a so called 'lecture', at this time a vaguely humorous and popular form of writing, printed in pamphlet form by Richard Braithwaite, he describes one woman thus:

the hair she wears comes from the periwig makers shop... her eyes have no other brows than those which a pencil makes nor her facer no other colour than that of painting... if she would suffer her face to be washed thou wouldst know her no more. She would be hideous unto thee... if thou wouldst kiss her all thy lips would be stuck with oil and grease.

His comments are very similar in nature and content to those of the satirical poets of the classical period. In the seventeenth century, just as the writers of ancient Greece and Rome had done, the woman is here, figuratively speaking, taken apart, bit by bit, to expose her true self; she has applied cosmetics to cover up the truth. Patches helped to disguise flaws in the complexion and a vizard might completely conceal a lady's face. The potential for mystery taking the most moral standpoint and deceit at the most immoral end of the scale was considerable. Men continued to be wary of such duping. There were even some quite practical solutions to finding out whether a woman was what she seemed. Men worried about being deceived might chew saffron and breathe on the woman. This would turn her make-up yellow if she was wearing any and did no harm to her complexion if she were not. I assume that if a lady's make-up that had been applied quite thickly, as was the fashion of the day and was slightly sticky, the yellow saffron would adhere to this. However, the option of such an experiment was only open to wealthy gentlemen as saffron was, and indeed remains, an expensive commodity.

Cosmetics and Murder

Around 1690 the story goes that one Signora Toffana began selling a product that may have been responsible for the deaths of as many as 600 people, mostly husbands whose wives wanted rid of them. The product she allegedly dispensed was either scented water, or perhaps a face powder, most frequently referred to as Aqua Toffana. Those who bought it were generally aggrieved wives who knew that they were buying an effective poison. These women were given strict instructions by Signora Toffana to apply this to their faces when there husbands were in the vicinity but to make sure they held their breath – a tall order. Aqua Toffana was supposed to have contained arsenic (a poison with no taint or odour which in past times had been difficult to detect) mixed with belladonna, a dangerous ingredient often used in eye cosmetics to create a dewy, large eyes impression. However this is only one version of the tale. Exactly who Signora Toffana was, and what the true facts of the case were, remain confused. However, the suggestion of death by make-up caused men in Italian society to be on their guard.

Sir Thomas Overbury was also believed to have been poisoned using make-up. The accused was one Mrs Anne Turner. The widow of a London doctor and a dressmaker by trade, Mrs Turner was also a well-known London purveyor of cosmetics and perfumes. Sir Thomas Overbury, who has been linked with those who eventually carried out the Gunpowder Plot, died in 1613 while he was locked up in the Tower of London. He had apparently been opposed to the Countess of Essex' proposed marriage to the Earl of Somerset and to keep him quiet, the Countess had allegedly employed Mrs Turner to silence him using a poison disguised as a cosmetic. This incriminating information did not catch the ear of King James I until two years after the murder took place. The said Anne Turner was duly found guilty at her trial in 1615 and hanged, but many others very close to the king were implicated – causing a national scandal. Once a favourite of the king, Robert Carr, Earl of Somerset, and Frances Howard his wife whose marriage plans had sparked the whole thing off were also condemned to death. However the couple were pardoned by the king and finally released from the Tower in 1622. This was a crime of passion and political intrigue with make-up, not for the first nor the last time, the means of execution. Both Jonson, with his character Mrs Turner and her 'oyle of talc' in his play *The Devil is an Ass,* and other writers, including Thomas Tuke in his book *A Discourse against Painting,* based their texts on the real-life scandal of the Overbury murder.

Branded Goods

Puppy dog water may have been even more unpleasant than one might at first suspect. One might think this is just another recipe using urine, in this case puppy urine, but the product does seem to have been a more gruesome mixture than that. According to Mary Doggett's *Book of Receipts* (1682) this was the distillation of the fat of an actual puppy killed for the purpose. The fat was mixed with a 'pint of fasting spittle in as quart of new buttermilk 2 quarts of white wine lemons acrimony and camphire'.

Bauer's head and bath soap is not quite what we imagine as soap, at least not in terms of its use. Made from rosemary, borax and glycerine, it was used to clean, strengthen and promote the growth of the hair as well as treating the skin. This was apparently a luxury product, exclusively manufactured by Osborne, Bauer & Cheeseman, perfumers to the Queen. Royal patronage was often claimed but not always genuine. The soap was also recommended as a shaving soap.

An advertisement for Robert Turner's dentifrice dated 1660 promises that it not only cleans the teeth, turning them as white as ivory, but also prevents toothache which, if it was an effective cleaner, would of course be logical. The dentifrice also fastens the teeth, sweetens the breath and preserve the mouth and gums. The manufacturer one Robert Turner describes himself in his advertisement as a gentleman. The outlet for his efficacious product is but one as was customary at this time; directions are given 'the right are only to be had at Thomas Rookes stationer at the holy lamb at the east end of St Pauls church near the school in sealed papers at 12d the paper'. He adds that 'The reader is desired to beware of counterfeits'. This caution became a sort of get out clause. It something went wrong and perhaps all the clients teeth remained stained or fell out, then Robert would be able to claim that in fact the product the client had used was not the genuine article.

Miscellaneous Recipes

A freckle remover:

> Take a little alum beaten small and temper amongst it a well brayed white of an egg, put it on a milde fire stirring it always about that it wax not hard and when it casteth up the scum then it is enough wherewith anoint the freckles the space of three days ; if you will defend your self that you get no freckles on the face, then anoint your face with the whites of eggs.
>
> Christopher Wirzung, *General practise of physicke*

To smooth rough and uneven skin:

> Take peeled almonds six pound, mastick prepared ceruse and gum dragant or each four ounces the whites of four eggs pound all together very carefully let it stand five or six days pounding it every day once then put them in a presse and keep the oil that comes forth to anoint the skin withall'
>
> Thomas Jeamson, *Artificial Embellishments*

To Beautifie the Face. Take cuckow-pintle a pretty quantity, bruise the thick parts with rosewater, dry them by the sun three or four days, then pouring more rose-water on it use it.

Hannah Woolley

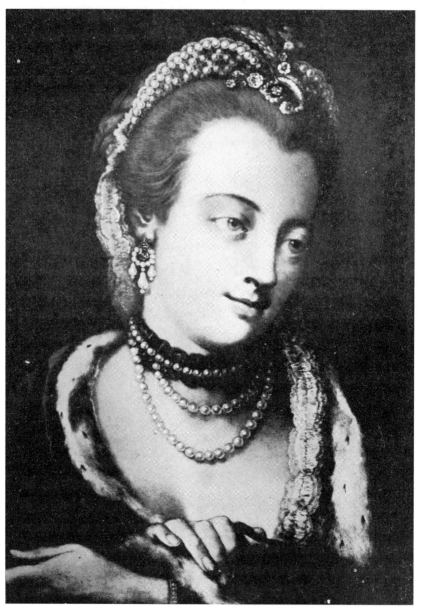

Maria Gunning from *A Georgian Pageant* (1908)

'Lady Coventry died at an early age with all her beauty gone and after suffering agonies from a cancerous disease of the face brought on by painting her cheeks'
The Hampshire Telegraph and Sussex Chronicle (1884)

6

THE EIGHTEENTH CENTURY:
COUNTERFEIT COSMETICS, THE FRENCH REVOLUTION, AND THE IMPORTANCE OF BEING SEEN

Fashion is the science of appearance, and it inspires one with the desire to seem rather than to be

Henry Fielding, author and playwright

Introduction

In the years prior to the French Revolution, which began in 1789, men and women, especially at the French court, wore a good deal of make-up. The effect was obvious and that was the intention. Not only was the French fashion of wearing make-up to excess adopted, by and large, by the rest of Europe but also the French language dictated the vocabulary relating to cosmetics in the eighteenth century. The term *cosmetique* referred to creams and make-up in general, while the word *fard* meant paint intended to cover imperfections, whether natural flaws, the ravages of disease, or the damage caused by the original application of the make-up itself. *Fard* was described as *blanc* or *rouge*, that is white or red, probably because these were dominant colours in use – a white foundation and a suitably noticeable application of red blusher.

Herbals, cookery books and etiquette books continued to carry recipes for all sorts of beauty products, just as they had done in the previous century. Increasing rates of literacy, especially among women, created an avid readership for these and for the flourishing market in a new medium, namely ladies magazines. Ingredients to make cosmetics were still bought to be put together at home but these homemade products now had to compete with an increasing number of goods manufactured outside the home in chemist shops and other small business outlets. Many of these commercial beauty products bore names intended to make them sound exotic and exclusive. Creams and potions were often credited with a deliberately mysterious provenance and exalted claims were made regarding their properties and effectiveness. Commercially produced luxury cosmetics were largely manufactured in France and initially imported into the capital cities of other European countries by individual men and women who had purchased these items as gifts for friends or lovers. However, due to the high demand for these goods, a more regular trade began to develop. If these French exotics were too expensive for one's pocket, then imitation goods could be purchased from chemists and perfumers shops or from itinerant street sellers at a cheaper price. In the eighteenth century, make-up had become affordable and, as a result, many were wearing it.

Every so often sumptuary legislation was passed in an effort to curb any tendency for personal excess. These laws were usually aimed at keeping a check on clothing or jewellery but, on occasion, included restrictions on cosmetics as well. The following text is from an Act of Parliament proposed in 1770:

All women, of whatever rank, profession or degree, whether virgins maids or widows that shall from and after such act, impose upon seduce and betray into matrimony any of his majesty's subjects by the scents paints, cosmetic washes, artificial teeth, false hair, Spanish wool, iron stays, hoops high heeled shoes and bolstered hips shall incur the penalty of the law now in force against witch craft and like misdemeanours and that the marriage upon conviction shall be null and void.

Despite its intention, this legislation was never enacted and in the end it was the political upheaval of the French Revolution that brought about a change in the way make-up was worn. The fashion for wearing heavy make-up was seen as one of the obvious excesses of the French court. So, although beauty products continued to be popular, after the revolution these were applied in a far more subtle manner in France itself and across Europe. Moderation in foundation and rouge was the key to a fashionable and, of no less significance, a respectable look. Suffice to say, in the last years of the eighteenth century the emphasis switched from ostentatious display to a concern for health and hygiene, with skin care assuming the upmost importance. Good hygiene increasingly necessitated the use of skin care products and cleansers as this more natural look became fashionable but bathing, although customary for medicinal purposes, was far from a daily routine at this time.

The Fashionable Woman

At the very beginning of the eighteenth century there was a brief and somewhat curious fashion for sporting a complexion of a rather unpleasant shade of green. The Scottish physician John Maubray remarks upon this in his work *The Female Physician* (1724): 'I have known', he says, 'many women in France and Germany who have been so far from thinking it [green] an ugly colour that they have esteemed it beautiful and have used very pernicious things to gain an appropriate colour for themselves.' More commonly a woman who was regarded as beautiful would possess the more traditional porcelain complexion, achieved very often through the application of a thick layer of white paint, with her lips either coloured red or left natural. Scented powders applied to the face helped make a lady look not only pale but exude a pleasant smell. Despite the fact that white lead had been officially declared a poison in the previous century, this was still being used in cosmetic preparations in the eighteenth century. However, the use of lead-based make-up was at least beginning to be called into question. According to an edition of *The Ladies Magazine* published in 1784; 'A little rouge is very pardonable but white paint is now looked on as disgraceful and dangerous.' Though the overall complexion was pale, colour was important and, as a result, rouge was very much in favour.

As far as other facial features were concerned the beautiful woman should possess dark, attractively curved eyebrows with little or no actual eye make-up. A woman's hair, whether black, blonde or brunette, should be topped off by a hair piece or perhaps completely covered by an elaborate wig. Red hair, popular in the days of Elizabeth I, was not highly thought of in the eighteenth century; still tarred perhaps by the connotations of witchcraft with which this colour had become associated in the seventeenth century. In fact, a woman with naturally red hair was likely, if she could, to hide it under a wig or to alter her natural hair colour with dye. To top it all off, hair powders for men as well as women were very much in vogue. According to the botanist Mary Frampton, in a diary entry for 1780, wearing hair powder was seen as a coming of age: 'I was dressed as a grown up for the first time and wore powder, the mark of distinction of womanhood'. Excess body hair remained an eyesore, especially when it came to women. The French chemist Nicholas Lemery in his work *Curiosa Arcana* (1711) recommends taking 'the shells of fifty-two eggs, beat them small and distil them with a good fire ... with the water anoint yourself where you would have the hair off'. The abrasive quality of the mixture may have removed tufts of hair but no doubt scraped and reddened the skin in the process.

Fashionable Men

Men, who were concerned about their appearance in the years before the French Revolution, wore elaborate wigs, darkened their eyebrows, applied rouge and might redden their lips. In Britain, very fashionable men were initially known as Macaronis and later as Dandies, Beau Brummell being the most well-known of these. The Italian name Macaroni came about because these fashionistas were often young men who had been on The Grand Tour of Europe, travelling abroad as part of their education. They adopted the fashions they found in other countries, bringing new ideas back with them from their travels and encouraging others to adopt alternative styles of dress. On account of their penchant for fashion, the Macaronis or Dandies found themselves subject to stinging criticism and ridicule. An edition of *Town and Country* magazine from 1764 reads; 'They [the Dandies] make a most ridiculous figure … it is a puzzle to determine the thing's sex.' However, derogatory comments like this do not appear to have deterred these young men from their enthusiasm for clothes and cosmetics. Although their appearance cast doubt on their suitability with regards to holding a public position in society, these gentlemen may have been too busy enjoying their leisure time to worry too much about that.

Some important male members of society, who did hold public office, followed the lead of the Macaronis and wore make-up. Lord John Hervey is an example of a man in an important position whose appearance was flamboyant. A courtier and English gentleman, he had acquired a liking for pale foundation when in Paris. In a statement in the same vein as the quotation from the *Town and Country* magazine above, Hervey's long-time friend, the well-travelled aristocrat Lady Mary Montagu (1689 –1762), remarked that 'the world consisted of men, women and Herveys'. In fact Hervey was drawn sexually to men and women and this is an early reference to what became known as the third sex.

However, it seems that Lord John did have poor health, perhaps even suffering for epilepsy. He may have worn make-up for a quite legitimate reason; that is, to conceal the physical evidence of his poor constitution.

Cosmetics and Counterfeits: The Importance of Authenticity

The burgeoning market in cosmetics led to fierce competition and to claim and counterclaim with regard to the benefits and advantages or disadvantages of specific products. The commercial market still had to compete with home-produced products but those trading in cosmetics had the opportunity, and the financial means, to push home the message through advertising that theirs was a superior product and was better manufactured. Although in its infancy, small discreet entries in newspapers promoting particular products were not uncommon. Some, for example, claimed their rouge would last many years, others that their product travelled well even in hot weather. Inventive claims added, no doubt, to the cachet of the product and subsequently the cost of purchasing it and might also have provided those who believed that make-up was trickery with ammunition by contradicting any claims made. Take for example, *Abdeker: The Art of Preserving Beauty* penned by Antoine le Camus, the head of the French faculty of medicine at the University of Paris in 1754. The text purports to be a translation of a manuscript written in Arabic, an illusion in itself which adds to the mystique of the book's content. Camus tempts his female audience with make-up described in mysterious terms, for example, 'a mixture of a spoonful of spirituous vulnerary [healing] water with two spoons full of river water'. According to Camus 'it preserves the complexion so French and fair that a woman of seventy after using it will look as if she was not above thirty-five'; effectively, an elixir of very unclear composition is offered with an extraordinary and no doubt tempting promise to women in Western society where youth was still regarded as an essential component of beauty.

One of the major concerns of those in the business of selling make-up was that there were always risks that their own product could be copied by others. The Widow Dupré, a supplier of rouge to the French court in the eighteenth century, notified her customers that: 'There is sold daily in Paris and in the provinces rouge marked and numbered as coming from my factory that can only harm my favourably established reputation seeing that these different sellers or makers falsify my rouge or make it themselves with harmful ingredients'. Widow Dupré even began to sign her packages personally in order to avoid counterfeits.

Packaging had been important as far back as Ancient Egyptian times. Elaborate containers were visible and tangible signs of the wealth and status of their owner. Expensive jars and bottles might also be taken as an indication of the nature or the quality of the product they contained, though this was not always accurate as vessels could be reused. In the eighteenth century the appearance of cosmetic bottles and boxes became important as a means of avoiding a less-effective and perhaps dangerous substitute for the real thing; luxury products came in quality bottles or boxes with elaborate labels and might even be signed as proof of authenticity.

Careful instructions about how to apply a product were often provided with the purchase. Some sellers and manufacturers might even pay a home visit to demonstrate the effective application of their make-up. However, if a cosmetic did not live up to the claims being made for it, then the seller might still argue that the user had not followed the instructions correctly. *Caveat emptor*, that is, 'buyer beware' was very much the watchword when it came to eighteenth century make-up, particularly if it were purchased rather than home produced. At this time, the consumer could claim no compensation, and had no comeback or redress if things went wrong.

A problem page in an early eighteenth century newspaper poses a further question that concerned many would-be husbands at the time: that is, had he married the woman he thought he had married? The article reads:

> No man was so enamoured as I was with her fair forehead neck and arms as well as the bright jet of her hair; but to my great astonishment I find they were all the effect of art. Her skin is so tarnished with this practice that when first she wakes in the morning she scarce seems young enough to be the mother of her whom I carried to bed the night before. I shall take the liberty to part with her by the first opportunity unless her father will make her portion suitable to her real not her assumed countenance.

Men feared being duped by the clever application of make-up.

Ladies were also worried about being deceived with regard to cosmetics. They sought out reputable sources and advice about their make-up to avoid at the very least a fashion *faux pas* and, at the extreme, damage to their skin or even internal organs through the use of harmful substances sold as being safe. Since scholarly medical texts continued to include cosmetics, believing them an important part of a health and hygiene regimen, women often sought advice from respectable medical practitioners whom they trusted to prescribe cosmetics that would do them no harm. These doctors were no doubt happy to cater for women (or men) who wanted their counsel as it brought them business and a steady income.

Make-up: To See and be Seen

Life at court involved a great deal of time just standing around waiting, hoping to be noticed most especially by the king or queen but also perhaps by other members of the royal family or other influential members of the aristocracy. The whole point of the exercise was to network and find favour with important people. One's appearance played a significant part in attracting that initial attention. In Britain, the tradition of the London Season, when all those of any wealth and social standing flocked to the city to engage with the rest of society, was well established by 1730. This was a stage for getting noticed beyond the regular court setting. An issue of *The Penny Magazine* from the later date of 1837 explains the original reasoning behind the timing of the London Season:

> The London 'season', or winter, was reckoned, during [the eighteenth century], from about the month of November till that of May. It was regulated...by the usual duration of the session of Parliament.

This event, or convention if you like, provided opportunities for arranging marriages (and thereby forging important political as well as social alliances), for moneymaking, and for generally enhancing one's social status. Attractive and fashionable women might find themselves in liaisons with men in powerful positions. Political ambitions could be advanced and secrets uncovered. There was considerable potential for an eighteenth-century scandal, similar to the Profumo affair that belongs in the twentieth century. Louis-Sébastien Mercier's renowned twelve-volume *Le Tableau de Paris* (published between 1781 to 1788), is a work that gives us much detail on what daily life in pre-revolutionary France was like; he remarks: 'Heavens! Get them to talk about the morning toilet and we would know state secrets.'

The London Season was indeed a grand opportunity for members of the upper classes in general to show themselves off to royalty and to each other but also to be seen in all their splendour by those who belonged to the lower classes too. Women, in particular, showed themselves off to the general public. They walked or rode in carriages up and down the stylish streets of the city while others, not only men but other women, looked on. Wearing make-up was essential for such a day of fashion. Street sellers or hawkers used the opportunity to sell their beauty products. In a satirical work entitled *St James Park* dating from 1733, a salesman offers: 'Pomatum my lady of all sorts, lip salves, forehead cloths, night masks, and handkerchiefs for her face and neck. Rich chemical liquor to change the colour of your hair and trotter oil and bears grease to thicken it'. Every opportunity was taken to sell these wares and there were plenty of buyers willing to spend their money.

Skin Care

Removing or concealing blemishes from spots to freckles continued to be a priority in the eighteenth century. A flawless pale skin was, as ever, the height of fashion, especially for women. In a letter written in 1762 to Lady Strangeways, Lady Bunbury notes: 'The Duchess of Grafton was there too and having left red and white quite off she is one of the coarsest brown women I ever saw'. This is not a comment about race but about status and about falling short of the expected standard of appearance.

It was not just the face that required attention. The arms, neck and bust were also painted to look pale. Chio Paste was one foundation used to whiten the skin at this time. This product, according to contemporary advertisements was, 'universally acknowledged' as 'kind to the skin and free from any injurious substances such as mercury'. Probably made from an aromatic resin, Chio Paste could be bought, especially in the latter part of the eighteenth century, in fashionable parts of London such as New Bond Street and Pall Mall and was even being sold at the post office in Chelsea. A newspaper article from 1791 quotes a price of

2s 6d for a pot. Full instructions were supplied for this price but no size or amount are given so it is not clear how much you got for your money.

Products to make the skin pale could still be made at home. Oliver Goldsmith (1728–1774) in his novel *The Vicar of Wakefield* paints a comical picture of just such an activity while at the same time hinting at the continued undercurrent of distrust of cosmetics that still existed at this time, despite their overt popularity. The eponymous vicar, Mr Charles Primrose, states,

> As we expected our landlord the next day my wife went to make the venison pasty … my daughters seemed equally busy … and I observed them for a while cooking something over the fire. I at first supposed they were assisting their mother; but little Dick informed me with a whisper that they were making a wash for the face. Washes of all kinds I had a natural antipathy to; for I knew that instead of mending the complexion they spoiled it. I therefore approached my chair by sly degrees to the fire and grasping the poker as if it wanted mending seemingly by accident overturned the whole composition and it was too late to begin another.

Despite our vicar's opinion, not all eighteenth century skin care products could be condemned out of hand as dangerous or harmful. A recipe for skin whitener from *The Toilet of Flora*, a popular title by a French doctor named Pierre-Joseph Buc'hoz, first published in 1779, reads as follows:

> Take equal parts of the root of centaury [cornflower] and the white vine, a pint of cow's milk and the crumb of a wheaten loaf; distil in a glass alembic [a piece of alchemical equipment used for distilling]. The distilled water for use must be mixed with an equal quantity of Hungary water [a distilled perfume

based on alcohol and rosemary]: it then admirably clears the complexion. The distilled waters of fennel and white lilies with a little gum mastic will produce the same effect.

The centaury gets its name from the legend that its effectiveness in healing skin was first discovered by the centaur and physician Chiron of Greek mythology. Nowadays fennel is known for its soothing properties in drinks as well as lotions. The benefits of fresh milk for dry skin had been known since at least the days of Cleopatra. There is nothing in this mixture to be concerned about. On the contrary, there were potential advantages in applying this.

Rouge

The blush was, as ever, a visibly readable sign of female modesty and considered a reliable reflection of good morals. A respectable woman was expected to blush, at the right time, and on the right occasion. Indeed, according to physician Dr John Gregory (1724–1771) in a conduct book entitled *A Father's Legacy to his Daughters* (1761), a work he wrote for his own daughters, 'when a girl ceases to blush, she has lost the most powerful charm of beauty'. Despite concerns that this sort of make-up had the potential to feign lost modesty, rouge, that artificial blush, was very fashionable. Vermillion, cochineal, safflower (a fatty acid now used as an ingredient in hair conditioners), saffron, gum resin, sandalwood (which has a strong smell) and brazilwood (which produces a warm brown tone) were all used as rouges in the eighteenth century. Mixed with lemon or vinegar or with powder (perhaps alum) and scented with a flower-based perfume, rouge could be applied easily and effectively with a brush. A rouge box, like a small mirror, might be carried about on one's person to repair one's complexion as necessary. Alternatively, a wet cloth or even a wet ribbon, dyed perhaps with cochineal, could be applied directly to the face to stain the cheeks red. Vermillion and sandalwood were both imported from the East Indies for use as rouge and as ever their exotic origins not only made them desirable but also inflated their price. However, while products like these may have been expensive, this did not necessarily make them a good long-term investment. Vermillion or cinnabar, that is mercuric sulphide, certainly imparted a very bright red to ladies' cheeks but was by no means a safe option as Abdeker (aka Albert Camus) makes clear:

> Cinnabar is composed of brimstone and mercury. When it is reduced to a subtle powder in a marble mortar it acquires so lovely and so high a colour that it is called vermillion. Some ladies mix it with paint herewith they rub their cheeks which is very dangerous for by using it frequently they may loose their teeth acquire a stinking breath and excite copious salivation.

The colours of the various materials used as rouge varied. Dye from the root of the plant alkanet was a safer option than vermillion or cinnabar if one wanted to sport a bright red shade of blusher. Aside from the bright red of vermillion or alkanet root, there was cochineal, also known as carmine, which was red with bluish tones, while minium or red lead, again a dangerous substance, produced more of an orange shade.

Eyes and Eyebrows

Little or no eye make-up was worn at this time but nicely curved eyebrows were in vogue. The juice of elderberries or burnt powder made from cork or cloves was used to draw in and accentuate one's brows. Fake brows were readily on sale and purchased by both men and women. These could be added to one's natural brows and glued on with mastic gum to hold them in place. However, false eyebrows were the focus of much derision. Take, for example, the following lines of satirical verse by poet and diplomat Matthew Prior written in 1718; 'If we don't catch a mouse tonight alas no eyebrows for tomorrow'. Given the genre (that is satire) and the fact that from a modern point of view, eyebrows made from mouse skin may seem more than a little odd, the reader might want to dismiss this as at best poetic licence or maybe simply as a joke. However Fairfax House, a Georgian townhouse (now a museum) in York's Castlegate, has had on display an example of this very thing, a mouse hair brow, reminding us that, although we must be wary, we should not to be too hasty and simply dismiss what may be hard to believe.

Hair

Wigs were popular in Britain and France, although they took longer to become part of Italian dress and fashion. Indeed 250 Italian noblemen initially signed a petition declaring that they would never wear them. Italian women were slow to adopt wigs too but by the end of the century there were hundreds of wigmakers working in the stylish city of Venice. Even the Italian men who had originally resisted wearing these items were persuaded to do so as it was only right and proper, indeed even a commercial advantage, for businessmen and dignitaries to meet their counterparts from abroad wearing the latest fashions.

In polite eighteenth century society, men wore full wigs while women tended to wear hair pieces to augment their own locks. Women also decorated their hair with everything from flowers to stuffed birds, even model ships in full sail. The expression 'big wig' has its origins in the idea that the bigger the wig, the more important the person. However according to author William Prynne (1600–1669), 'men who wear false hair or periwigs doe and doe commonly affirmed and sweare them to be their owne, (perhaps upon this evasion that they have paid well for them) and would have all men deeme them their natural and native haire'.

Hair to make lavish wigs was imported into the fashionable centres of Italy, France and Britain, from Parma, Tuscany and Belgium. The poor sold their own hair to traders at local fairs and markets to make wigs for the upper classes. Real hair was supplemented with unwashed sheep's wool, goat's hair or horsehair, all of which were, of course, highly flammable. While the use of animal hair in wigs was illegal, it was quite common in practice as it could take up to ten heads of hair to make a man's full bottomed wig. Wool, however, was recognised as legitimate wig-making material. Although the expression 'to pull the wool over someone's eyes' does not appear until the nineteenth century it may have its origin in the wool wigs worn by judges when these slipped over their eyes, perhaps falling asleep, and they could potentially be deceived by the convicted man or woman before him. While a wig was easier to clean and maintain in some ways, there was always the worry that one had bought hair that was infected with a serious disease. Pepys notes this concern when writing in his diary in 1665; 'Nobody', he says, 'will dare buy a hair for fear of infection that it has been cut off the heads of people dead of the plague'. Pepys also points out that wigs were not necessarily free from unpleasant infestations either. He explains that he himself has encountered this problem; 'I did go to the Swan; and there sent for Jervas my old periwig maker and he did bring me a periwig but it was full of nits ... and did send it back to make it clean.' Nevertheless it was probably a simpler matter to get your wig deloused by another than to have to try to rid your own hair of an infestation in the eighteenth century. Sometimes the height of the coiffure created other pressing practical problems. In order to travel in their carriages, ladies might have sit on the floor. Sleeping could also be an issue. Elaborate styles might require the wearer to spend the night propped up, their hair sometimes covered with a large hood, hardly a prescription for a good night's sleep. However, we should not be too influenced by the cartoons and caricatures of ladies and gentlemen sporting tall wigs that appeared frequently in publication at this time; by their very nature these images do exaggerate reality. At any rate, by the middle of the century, easy to wear wigs were becoming more common. Men who belonged to the social elite adopted styles originally worn by the professional classes, (such as the rather looser and more informal bagwig) rather than aristocratic or court styles that were standard in the earlier part of the eighteenth century. This change was brought about largely by practical considerations including the cost of the more elaborate wig as well as the problems posed, such as the weather and for greater convenience of movement and travel. By the end of the century. less ostentatious styles were more likely to be worn on a day-to-day basis by women too – both for practical reasons similar to those that had encouraged men to adopt these styles and as a reaction to the excesses of the revolution in France.

A Visit to the Hairdressers

Both men and women might visit the barbers. An entry in the diary of James Woodeforde, a country parson, reads: 'Nancy [his niece] walked with me to one Smiths in Surrey Street The Strand. A barber and there had her hair fully dressed. I was shaved and had my wig fully dressed there'. It was not unusual for a woman to have hair styled at such an establishment, although she would not have had her locks washed or cut. James Woodeforde doesn't tell us whether his niece was wearing a wig. Perhaps he was being discreet. Professional hairdressers attended public events and venues too. Ladies were alerted accordingly through adverts in newspapers. The following notice appeared in the *Salisbury and Winchester Journal* in July 1786:

> Woolard, Hairdresser, Fountain Buildings Bath, begs leave most respectfully to acquaint the Nobility and Gentry that he

will attend to dress at the following places: Winchester Races and Music Meeting; Salisbury Races and Music Meeting; and Blandford Races; Those Ladies who please to honour him with their commands, (which are requested to be in writing, to prevent mistakes) at the Royal Oak Inn, High street, Winchester; Mr. Hill's, shoemaker, High street, Salisbury; and the Blue Boar Inn, Blandford, will be punctually attended.

By all accounts a lady could combine a day's outing with her husband to a social event such as the races or a music recital with having her hair done.

Hair Powders and Pomatums

From the turn of the century, hair powders were used extensively by men and women. Rather in the manner of a dry shampoo, the powder removed some of the dirt and grease. However this was not its only purpose. Louis XIV, King of France, did so to cover his thinning hair. His courtiers old and young followed his example and it became common practice to powder one's wig too. In an entry in her journal in 1779, the diarist and botanist Mary Frampton gives the following description of the cosmetic treatment of hair:

I insert this trivial remark and message to myself to mark the fashion of the times when all gentlemen wore queues, or tails of considerable length and thickness near the head, dwindling by degrees towards the extremity, with a little bow of ribbon near the head, and a small brush of hair at the end, the whole well-plaistered and powdered, and great curls frizzed, powdered and pomatumed at the ears, called sometimes canons from their shape. The ladies wore the hair flowing down their backs and high in front, with much pomatum and powder put on with different kinds of puffs. The finishing powder had a brown hue and a strong/perfumed smell, and was called 'Marechale' powder. This powder was applied at a distance, that every hair might be frosted with it. One pound, and even two pounds, of powder were sometimes put into the hair or wasted in the room in one dressing.

Frampton describes a lengthy and elaborate process involving the use of copious amounts of powder to achieve the desired ostentatious, and no doubt, striking effect. Pomatum, a greasy substance made from lard or animal fat (often bear fat), was applied to the hair to control the style. A mix of water, almond oil or beeswax also doubled as the basis of face cream. Pomatum derives its name from the fact that these ointments were originally scented with apple (in Latin *poma*). To appeal to potential users, pomatum was scented, perhaps with lemon or orange; to be more specific, bergamot, an oily substance obtained from a small variety of Seville orange. The author John Galsworthy in his novel The *Country House* (1907) remarks upon the pungent and long-lasting nature of this greasy hair perfume. 'A footman and a groom came next, leaving trails of pomatum in the air.' Clearly if someone was wearing it, the odour was all-pervasive. At a large gathering of the well-to-do one could imagine that the mingling smells of pomatums of different scents must have been quite overpowering. Although Galsworthy's novel was written at a much later date than the period under discussion here and the setting for his story also postdates the eighteenth century, it seems reasonable to imagine that in the eighteenth century a similar strong smell of hair perfume pervaded wealthy country homes and town houses.

Hair powders were made from wheat flour or sieved starch and scented with violet, orris root (which has a similar odour to violet), or perhaps with the strong aromatic odour of civet, derived from the anal glands of members of the cat family. Almond powder, basically residue of almonds or the crumbs from the bottom of the packet as it were, was one cheap option. Hair powder was usually white but could be tinted violet or pink, or even brown as in the case of Marechale powder mentioned by Miss Frampton. The exact composition of Marechale powder is unknown though given its colour, this may have included cinnamon or perhaps mace. Powdered white lead was also used on hair and even gold dust might be worn by the wealthy. When applied to dark hair the effect of the more common white hair powder was greying, though on blonde hair this could lighten the locks and therefore conceal any grey. Again, according to Mary Frampton writing in her diary in 1780, 'Everybody wore powder and pomatum.' These powders were blown onto the hair with a set of bellows. To avoid covering the face as well and getting the powder in their eyes, the lady or gentleman held up a paper cone in front of her face to shield it from harm in a not dissimilar fashion to a woman at a hairdressers today protecting her face with a paper mask from an application of hair spray. The wealthy might set aside a small room in their grand house for this purpose, preventing the powder covering good furniture elsewhere in the house.

The walls of great houses were decorated with canvases that show their owners in all their finery, including their powdered wigs. These paintings were one way of impressing one's visitors and reinforcing the social standing of the owners of property that they had just entered. For us they are a visual record of the fashions of the times. The painting of the Ladies Waldegrave, sisters Anne, Charlotte and Elizabeth, dates from 1783 and now hangs in the National Art Gallery in Edinburgh. Originally the canvas would have graced the walls at the family home at Ragley Hall, Alchester, near Warwick. The hair appears grey, the result of the use of hair powder. As dry as tinder, these headdresses were easily set alight and the fashion for powdered hair in high styles continued to prove a health and safety hazard. The wigs or hairpieces worn by women at court, particularly on special occasions, were tall and ornate and were liable to get caught in chandeliers, setting fire to the hair, causing severe burns and even, on occasion death. The grease and powder in the wigs worn by aristocratic ladies are edible substances and so provided a breeding ground of lice and other vermin, making a scratching stick not only a fashion accessory but rather a necessity. The popularity of hair powder faded when William Pitt the Younger imposed stamp duty on packets of hair powder in 1786 and subsequently, in 1795, passed a law banning its use on wigs without a licence.

Lips and Teeth

Lipstick took rather a back seat in terms of fashion in the eighteenth century. In France the same substances used as rouge were applied to redden lips. Simply pinching the lips to make them bleed and therefore redden, or rubbing them with lemon juice, could produce the desired effect if one was in a hurry. The lips could equally be left unadorned. However attention was paid to teeth. Teeth from conflicts, including the battlefields in Spain and the rout of the Jacobites in Scotland, quickly found their way to the dentists in cities like London and into the mouths of the well to do. Collecting live teeth from the battlefield may have been rather a gruesome trade but the financial rewards could be considerable; they fetched a good price. George Washington's dentist John Greenwood advertised for 'Live teeth ... for which a Guinea each will be given'. Sets of false teeth were also made from ivory and porcelain. The eccentric Lord John Hervey even had false teeth made from mottled brown jasper, though it is hard to imagine that these could have looked either clean or attractive.

Alternatively, one might try a product to improve the appearance of one's teeth and to counteract any infections or toothache. *The Pharmacopeia of Madrid*, dated 1739, records toothpowder made from powdered pumice stone, cuttlefish, cream of tartar, dragon's blood, red coral and orris root. Orris root is still sold at chemists as an effective herbal and natural treatment for toothache. The abrasive qualities of cuttlefish bone and pumice stone were well known in the ancient world and probably served their purpose. Spirit of vitriol or sulphuric acid was used to clean teeth but over time stripped off the surface enamel. A mixture of cloves, cinnamon, bramble leaves and honey mixed with burnt ashes sweetened the breath, in the short term at least. Parsley could be chewed to freshen breath and is still to be found in products to alleviate bad breath in animals today.

Maria Gunning: Death by Cosmetics

Maria Gunning was an Irish beauty of modest upbringing whose looks afforded her a good marriage to the 6th Earl of Coventry. She and her younger sister Elizabeth took London society by storm. They were the talk of the 1752 London Season, becoming known as 'the beauties'. Their comparatively meagre financial means proved no hindrance as it seems their looks more than made up for this shortcoming. The ladies were the celebrities of their day, needing an escort to keep the crowds, who wanted to admire their beauty, at a manageable distance. The distinguished author and Member of Parliament Horace Walpole declared the sisters 'the handsomest women alive'.

No doubt her notoriety brought Maria to the attention of the Earl of Coventry. When she visited Paris on honeymoon with her new husband, the countess developed an obsession with cosmetics. She seems to have had a particular liking for Venetian ceruse. A white powdered mixture produced by steeping lead in vinegar, (in essence the same product that women in the ancient world had used to whiten their complexion more than a thousand years earlier) this was one of the most popular skin lightening cosmetics worn by upper-class fashion-conscious women of the eighteenth century. The initial effect was of a white opaque finish. Before long, however, this make-up corroded the skin, often resulting in more and more being applied to hide the damage already done.

Prolonged exposure to ceruse is now known to cause mental deterioration, hair loss, muscle paralysis and even damage to internal organs. At least some of the dangers of using lead-based make-up were known in the eighteenth century, as they had been to the Greeks and Romans. It is probable these ill effects were common knowledge, though it does not seem to have put women off using such products. In the end Maria's excessive use of dangerous make-up, and white lead in particular, allegedly caused her death at the age of just twenty-seven in 1760. According to the newspapers of the day, she was a 'victim of cosmetics' although some form of consumptive disease probably also contributed to her early demise. In death Maria continued to fascinate. Thousands came to the funeral to view her coffin.

The countess's legendary beauty is preserved in the many portraits painted of her. While those by Sir Joshua Reynolds are not considered to be his best work, the most admired works were painted by Francis Cotes, a founding member of The Royal Academy. In 1884, more than 100 years after her death, *The Hampshire Telegraph and Sussex Chronicle* refers to Maria's untimely death in an effort to highlight the perils of applying cosmetics:

> Lady Coventry died at an early age with all her beauty gone and after suffering agonies from a cancerous disease of the face brought on by painting her cheeks ... when the late hours and bad air had destroyed the bloom which Maria Gunning had brought from her Irish hills and dales she endeavoured to replace it by the use of cosmetics with fatal effect ... It was a high price to pay for a little fleeting admiration.

In 2012 a mirror belonging to the countess sold at auction for £300,000. The over mantel mirror, some 7 feet in height, was made for her in 1759, the year before her death, so we can imagine that as she stood before it Maria must have had mixed feelings about the reflection of decaying beauty she saw reflected in the glass. Horace Walpole noted that 'Lady Fortose ... is at the point of death killed like Lady Coventry and others by white lead of which nothing could break her.' This was a sort of addiction. Clearly Lady Coventry was far from the only victim of this dangerous cosmetic practice. According to Hugh Walpole the courtesan Kitty Fisher, remembered in the children's nursery rhyme, also died as a result of her use of cosmetics. However this may be a conflation with evidence of the death of Maria Gunning the Countess of Coventry, her contemporary and her rival.

Trendsetters

Marie Antoinette, Queen of France, is credited with a recipe for a face mask made from cognac, egg, dry milk powder and the juice of a lemon. The make-up she is alleged to have worn is an extension of the criticism of her personality. Her ostentatious hairstyle was composed of a 3-foot-high wig built up with wire, gauze and cloth. This was powdered with white flour, and decorated with flowers, feathers, even vegetables and model ships. On a woman who was probably not very tall (she is described as not tall or of medium height in the contemporary sources) and bearing in mind that people in the eighteenth century were, on average, rather short, shorter indeed than they had been in medieval times, a 3-foot-high wig would have made movement awkward, potentially affecting her balance, especially when so many items were suspended in it, so the height is probably an exaggeration. Leonard Alexis Autier was employed as Marie Antoinette's hairdresser. He was the man responsible for these huge hairstyles but although he wrote his memoirs, these are more fiction than fact and as a result give us little useful information. However, it was her unnecessary use of white flour, a basic and essential food commodity, as hair powder that really got up the noses of the Paris mob. Marie Antoinette is alleged to have maintained her standards in terms of cosmetics right up to her demise at the guillotine, applying rouge to her cheeks when being given the last rites.

Other important ladies of the time were also renowned for their use of make-up. For example, Queen Anne used cosmetics lavishly and if she did, the ladies of her court would not be far behind. Georgiana, Countess of Devonshire, a member of the Spencer family and a great-great-great-great-aunt of Diana, Princess of Wales, wore very high wigs with ornaments such as stuffed birds, used a scratching rod and slept sitting up. Napoleon's valet describes Pauline Borgese, the sister of Napoleon thus: 'Nothing was lacking to her but a little youth for the skin of her face was beginning to be wrinkled, but the few defects which resulted from age disappeared under light coating of cosmetics which gave more animation to her pretty features'. Her lavish travelling case, containing numerous containers (some of these would have contained her make-up) can be seen on display in the National Museum of Scotland. Madame de Pompadour, mistress, of King Louis XV of France from 1745 to 1751 and an influential member of the French court, is painted (applying her make-up) on the canvas by Boucher with the same materials she would have applied as cosmetics on herself. The detail in the picture shows a period dressing table with powder puff to hand.

Trailblazers

Mary Wollstonecraft, writer and champion of women's rights, was hardly typical of women in the eighteenth century but in 1787 in 'Thoughts on the Education of Daughters' Mary expressed her belief that women's enthusiasm for cosmetics did not reflect well on the female character. She states:

On the article dress may be included the whole tribe of beauty washes cosmetics Olympian dew oriental herbs liquid bloom and the paint which enlivened Ninons face and bid defence to time these numerous and essential articles are advertised in so ridiculous a style that the rapid sale of them is a very severe reflection on the understanding of those females who encourage it.

The dew and herbs, I imagine, are very harmless but I do not know whether the same may be said of the paint. Pamphleteer, journalist and Member of Parliament, William Cobbett (1763 –1835), believed that women should not read about or be involved in politics at all and chooses Mary as an example of what might happen if a woman did take an interest in such things. It is, he says, 'well known that when that political lady began the rights of women she had as fine black hair as you would wish to see and that before her second week of her work went to the press it was turned as white and a great deal whiter than her skin'. Even if there is any truth in this anecdote, the likelihood is that Mary powdered her hair on occasion, which could make it look white or grey. There are portraits of her both with and without hair powder. Cobbett's assessment is ridiculous.

Lady Mary Wortley Montagu (1689–1762) had a rather more worthy connection with make-up. Mary was a smallpox survivor. The disease had disfigured her so much she used cosmetics to conceal the scars. In 1740 Horace Walpole described Lady Montagu's complexion in the following unflattering manner: 'Her face swelled violently on one side with the remains of the pox partly covered with a plaister and partly with white paint which for cheapness she had bought so coarse that you would not use it to wash a chimney'. No doubt she had every reason for wanting to use cosmetics to cover up the damage done by disease. Mary travelled abroad with her husband, an ambassador to the court of Turkey and a representative of the Levant Company. Her letters published the year after her death reveals her fascination with the beauty and the lack of inhibition of women in Turkey. Lady Mary expresses in her letters much appreciation for the welcoming reception she received from other women in Turkey:

> I know no European court where the ladies would have behaved themselves in so polite a manner to a stranger. I believe in the whole there were two hundred women and yet not one of these disdainful looks or satiric whispers that never fail in our assemblies when any body appears that is not dressed exactly in fashion.

Her comments reflect both the competition in looks and fashion that could turn nasty at court, as well as the importance of etiquette and conformity in Europe at this time. It is Lady Mary Montagu's role in instituting routine smallpox vaccinations to avoid the damage to appearance that she herself had suffered that had important and lasting legacy. Lady Mary advocated administering a live vaccine against the disease to children, a practice she had witnessed firsthand on her travels.

However her own use of make-up was not always a positive experience for her. In fact, Mary seems to have been unlucky in her choice of products, trying various sorts of cosmetics in her travels and sometimes suffering the consequences. Her comments on Balm of Mecca, a scarce aromatic resin, show that despite its alleged benefits it affected her very badly and no doubt had the potential to affect others in the same way. She writes:

> The next morning, the change indeed was wonderful; my face was swelled to a very extraordinary size, and all over as red as my lady H's. It remained in this tormentable state three days, during which you may be sure I passed my time very ill. I believed it never would be otherwise; and to add to my

misfortune, Mr. W reproached my adventure without ceasing. However, my face is since in status quo; nay, I am told by the ladies here that it is much mended by the operation, which I confess I cannot perceive in my looking-glass. Indeed, if one was to form an opinion of this balm from their faces, one should think very well of it. They all make use of it, and have the loveliest bloom in the world. For my part I never intend to endure the pain of it again; let my complexion take its natural course, and decay in its own due time.

Mocking Make-up

By the end of the eighteenth century poking fun at make-up had become almost a pastime. Jonathan Swift (1667–1745), well known for his book *Gulliver's Travels,* joked,

> Here gallypots and vials placed,
> Some filled with washes, some with paste,
> Some with pomatum, paints and slops
> And ointments good for scabby chops.

A cleric as well as a writer, poet and pamphleteer, no doubt his religious beliefs influenced his attitude to cosmetics, but he was far from alone in expressing his opinions in this way. Cartoons mocking make-up were scathing and did not hold back. Lady Mary Archer, an eighteenth-century gambler renowned for her reliance on heavy make-up, was a subject lampooned in a series of contemporary cartoons. She was a woman, it has to be said, who laid herself open to abuse on account of her inability to stick to society etiquette. Independent (and once widowed, even more so), and a woman of expensive tastes, she openly gambled, playing a game of chance called Faro, and could be seen out and about in the company of men (often much younger than herself). In cartoon form, she suffered abuse that seems more hurtful than a few unkind words.

Even *The Lady's Magazine*, a publication clearly intended for a female audience, did not baulk at mocking women on the grounds of their appearance. In an edition published in 1777 the following rhyme appeared:

> Give Chloe a bushel of horsehair and wool,
> of paste and pomatum a pound,
> ten yards of gay ribbon to deck her sweet scull,
> and gauze to encompass it round,
> Let her gown be tucked up to the hip on each side,
> shoes too high for to walk or to jump,
> and to deck sweet charmer complete for a bride,
> let the cork cutter make her a rump,
> Thus finished in taste while on Chloe you gaze,
> You may take the dear charmer for life
> but never undress her, for out of her stays
> you'll find you have lost half your wife.

Perhaps this was an opportunity for women to be cruel to each other and vie with each other, eighteenth century style; an indication perhaps of the unpleasantness which Lady Mary Montagu had hinted at in her letters.

An edition of *The British Magazine and Review* also known as *Universal Miscellany of Arts and Sciences* dated 1783 observes:

> See gay Mrs. Tonith of Grosvenor Place
> How charmingly she enamels her face!
> She pencils in veins with azure blue;
> With black her eyebrows; combs them, too;
> She paints so true,
> In nature's hue,
> With red and white, amid Olympian dew,
> As makes her look like a doll quite new,
> And shoots macaroni's through and through.

While again this is pure satire, there are always some clues as to eighteenth-century fashions in make-up to be drawn from passages like this. This piece alludes to the practice of drawing blue veins on pale skin as well as to the burgeoning fashion for enamelling the face, a process that not only harks back to the Renaissance period when women coated their faces with egg white but alsolooks forward to the next century when so-called enamelling was championed by cosmetic practitioners and endorsed by those at the top level in society, including royalty. The passage also mentions one of the popular products of the day, that is, Olympian Dew, which in its name conjures up the illusion of the beauties of the classical world.

Popular Products

Let us start with that Olympian Dew referred to in rather unkindly fashion in the above article. *The New Family Receipt Book* (1837) gives a more favourable account of its properties:

> To the ladies Olympian Dew is recommended being the only thing discovered that will effectually clear the skin of freckles, pimples, tan and every deformity, it instantly makes wrinkles disappear and gives a loveliness to the countenance too charming to be described.

Olympian Dew, or Grecian Bloom as it was also known, was a multi-purpose product recommended to women for eradicating pimples, freckles and even wrinkles and marketed as a soothing aftershave for gentlemen. In 1786, according to newspaper advertisements, Olympian Dew was also a valued handkerchief perfume, endorsed by no less a person than Marie Antoinette herself; 'no perfume so sweet so delicate so refreshing as Olympian Dew says the Queen of France, she not only uses it herself but has commanded all her attendant nobility to do the same.' There was no comeback or legal penalty for claiming in print the backing of some person or persons of note if these claims were untrue, so this is a ploy used in many early advertisements. Olympian Dew was probably a skin tonic or scented water but its exact ingredients remain uncertain.

Princess Royal Powder was fragrant powder for the hair. An edition of *The Times* newspaper for 20 February 1786 carried a small and discreet advertisement for this hair powder that reads,

> to ladies of fashion the above powder was allowed to be the most fashionable and becoming on her majesty's birthday. It gives a richness and elegance to the hair hitherto unknown and possesses a fragrance of the most balsamic kind which renders it not only the most vivifying but the most fabulous powder and perfume ever used.

The advertisement goes on to state a price of 16s a pound and make clear that this exclusive product is only available from H. Dowling, Princes Street, London. It was also alleged that this was applied by Madame de Montespan, the mistress of the French king, Louis XIV. The mention of a connection with royalty would not go amiss in selling the product. The claim that this powder was the best and the latest thing is a common one made for many cosmetics at this time. *The Gazette of Health* advertises Bloom of Ninon de L'Enclos as follows:

> On examining this unequalled and inestimable cosmetic, we find it to be composed of white lead, almond emulsion, and essence of lavender. Now of all the compositions that have been offered to the public as cosmetics, this is the most dangerous. The repeated application of lead to the skin of the face, instead of animating the countenance, would assuredly, by paralysing the nerves, render it inanimate. Such are the baneful effects of lead on the constitution, that the most serious consequences have followed, even the partial use

of a weak preparation. What then must be the effect of the repeated application of a lotion strongly impregnated with it?

Bloom of Ninon was named after a French courtesan and patron, Ninon de L'Enclos. Its effect was to paralyse the nerves similar to modern-day Botox. But as we have seen the effects of white lead could be extensive and even fatal.

First produced in 1789, Pears soap was sold exclusively to his customers by its inventor Andrew Pears, a barber by trade. The soap was intended to improve the complexion and to counteract the roughness and damage done to the skin by toxic lead cosmetics. The soap, with its distinctive transparency, was produced by dissolving ordinary soap in alcohol, and distilling this to remove the alcohol. This process resulted in a clear jelly, which was then hardened in moulds.

A skin cream known as Denmark Lotion was made from bean flour, the juice of pomion (a variety of pumpkin), melon, cucumber and gourd. This was mixed with fresh cream and milk and as a result probably had to be used as used as soon as it was made up. The ingredients are certainly harmless and may, from a modern perspective, have merit. Pumpkin is a good source of fatty oil and antioxidants, the benefits of milk-based products had been well known for centuries, melon extract is now used in shampoos for dry hair, and cucumber is applied as a skin soother, especially around the eyes.

According to an advertisement for the attention of the ladies that appeared in the *The Times* in April 1788, Sharp's Sweet Cypress Hair Powder 'is the lightest sweetest and the best for the hair of any at 1s 2d per pound. Stamp included or 11s per dozen'. The advertisement also states that Sharps as a company 'supply all sorts of hair powder made (as may be seen every day) from the purest French starch and sold cheaper than any other house'. The seller is clearly at pains to stress the efficacy and the superior quality of this product mentioning French origins and the fact that the powder is made to order in front of the purchaser. A competitive price is an indication of the buoyant market in make-up at the time.

According to *Mists Weekly Journal* (1725):

At the Dove and Golden Ball in Salisbury Court, Fleet Street, liveth a Gentlewoman that prepares the most excellent Cosmetick or Beautifiers yet known, as that most noble Preparation of Pearl, with a particular beautifying Fluid, both which used by Ladies of the first Quality; They, with Surprize, take away Redness, Pimples, Roughness, Worms, Morphew, Scurf, Sunburn, Freckles, Wrinkles, Pits of the Smallpox, with other Defilements of the Skin. Likewise she prepares a fine Italian Cream for the Face Neck and Hands, which plumps and smoothes the Skin to Admiration; the Nuns White Pots, and Tower Street Pots, with an East India Chinese Red Liquor, none having the Secret but herself: It gives a most natural and lasting Blush, that no Person can distinguish when on the Face, and not to be rubbed off. Also to be had, the red Crown Cakes, White Paste, or Cakes for the face, or Hands, and all other Cosmeticks formerly sold here by Mrs. Hodde. N.B. She has chemical Liquor which alters red or grey Hair to a light or dark Brown'

Here is someone who is ahead of her time, making a large range of beauty products. Even at the beginning of the twentieth century, most cosmetic companies started off making either one single product or a very small range of items. This gentlewoman in her advertising promotion also recalls the past, alluding to her 'secrets', like those closely guarded by the alchemists of the fifteenth and sixteenth centuries, that make her products exclusive.

7

THE NINETEENTH CENTURY:
THE VICTORIANS, LADIES' MAGAZINES, CRIME AND COSMETICS

What could be prettier in a daintily decorated chamber than the richly draped toilet table with its glitter and sparkle of silver and crystal appointments – its air of refinement and luxury so dear to the heart of every true woman?

The Decorator and Furnisher (1896)

Introduction

At the beginning of the nineteenth century the Napoleonic Wars raged between the French under Napoleon and an assortment of other European countries. Inevitably, this confrontation had its effect on trade, causing, among other deprivations, a shortage of cosmetics, especially those products imported from the fashionable Italian city of Venice and from the East. In Britain, the long reign of Queen Victoria imposed one woman's ideas on self-presentation. For much of that time, Victoria was in mourning for her beloved husband Prince Albert and, as a result, fashions were sombre and reserved. Proper etiquette was more than ever creating a society with a stiff, prudish veneer, albeit contrasted with a much less virtuous underbelly. In polite society, a wife called husband Mr and he referred to her as Mrs. Such strict codes of behaviour influenced styles of dress including make-up. Manuals with instructions on etiquette and good manners, for ladies in particular, abound from this period with titles such as *The Young Woman's Companion* (1820), *The Book of Health and Beauty* or *The Toilette of Rank and Fashion* (1837) and *Beauty; Its Attainment and Preservation* (1892). The fact that so much emphasis was placed on advice about appearance in these manuals is made very clear even if one simply scans the titles.

At the beginning of the nineteenth century cosmetics were still, in the main, produced at home but by the middle of the century many more were shop bought. The Great Exhibition of 1851 was of considerable importance in putting on display what could be purchased for the purposes of enhancing one's appearance if one had the money to acquire such commodities. The rise of the department store selling beauty products on a day-to-day basis followed on from this popular and influential exhibition event. Not all make-up was expensive and cheap alternatives to the luxury cosmetics on sale and display at the Great Exhibition, for example, came in the form of mass-produced goods that the industrialised nations were now able to generate. These goods became readily available to the general public with less money to spend. Also, new beauty products, and ideas about how to wear these, began to arrive in Europe from a new commercial market, namely the United States of America.

As a consequence of a more readily available range of cheaper goods, the use of cosmetics became widespread. The writer, illustrator and member of the Dress Reform Society, Mary Haweis, in her book, *The Art of Beauty* first published in 1878 stated that; 'it is not wicked to take pains with oneself'. In earlier centuries there had been quite a trend for believing that it was indeed wicked to do exactly that. By the end of the nineteenth century, in 1895 in fact, *The London Journal of Fashions* could confidently state, 'the entirely unaided face is becoming rarer. Almost everybody uses other make-up effects if not rouge and almost scarlet lip salve.' Despite the reality of a more liberal and accepting approach to wearing cosmetics, the practice still drew considerable criticism from some – and not only from men, but from some women too. Lady Colin Campbell, an aristocratic and forward looking lady in other respects, was much opposed to make-up – condemning what she described in her book entitled *The Ladies Dressing Room* published in 1892 as ladies' 'deplorable and unbecoming mania for painting themselves'.

The Ideal Woman

Although the use of cosmetics was on the increase at all levels of society, in polite society at least, women and men still admired what was considered to be the natural look. A rather disturbing pale, fragile, almost sickly appearance, rather than a face that was highly coloured, was in fashion, one that could be compared not only with the green colouring that was briefly popular at the beginning of the eighteenth century but also with twentieth century 'heroin chic' that became trendy on the catwalks in the 1970s and '80s. Rouge was still widely used, though on the whole, bright colours were considered vulgar. Obvious make-up was deemed more suitable for the stage. Sadly, this fashion for the overly pale sickly look in the nineteenth century may have been counterproductive in terms of the projected view of women in general, serving to characterize them as the weaker sex, often in poor health, addicted to substances such as laudanum, and in temperament somewhat hysterical.

The use of skin care products, as distinct from paint (mainly foundation and rouge), became increasingly popular as the complexion continued to be taken as an indication of health and status, which any obvious use of cosmetics might be said to conceal or at best confuse. In 1879 the invention of the electric light bulb brought a new challenge for women who wore make-up; that is, how to look good in artificial light. Harriet Hubbard Ayer, the owner of the American make-up company Recamier, specifically included make-up intended to look good in electric light among the products she sold. Ayer comments,

> This would suit the society lady who at night might dine with friends or attend an opera or a ball in artificial light. At night before dinner as well as for the opera and ball, the artificial light makes it possible for a woman to literally put on her war paint and the make-up here suggested is intended for evening and to bear the glare of electric lights.

Ayer goes on to give a recipe for a white liquid that dried to a powder that should then be applied by one's maid to the face, neck and arms. This consisted of water, alcohol, oxide of zinc, mercury and glycerine. The exact measurements are given as one quart, thirty drops, one ounce, eight grains and twenty drops respectively. Suffice to say that although in the early years of the twentieth century, the use of artificial light in homes of the wealthy as well as in public places such as theatres and concert halls would become more widespread, in the latter years of the nineteenth century there was already an understanding that to make the best impression, make-up needed adjusting to suit the light, whether it be natural or artificial. This was especially important as one was more likely to encounter artificial light in public places where others would have the opportunity to scrutinise your appearance.

Men and Make-up

Chemist John Scoffern (1814–1882) expressed the opinion that 'cosmetics so they may be innocent are very appropriate for the fair sex but mostly stupid for men'. In general, men had in fact given up the rouge and powder that they had relied on in much of the seventeenth and eighteenth centuries. Indeed at the turn of the century, although Prime Minister William Pitt the Younger had repealed the law that decreed stamp duty was due to be paid on hair powder, perfume and cosmetics, a licence to use hair powder was required up until 1868. As hair powder was no longer profitable, its use declined. However, gentlemen in this the nineteenth century did spend money on certain hair products – being partial, in particular, to oils and dyes. Men made use of Buckingham's dye to hide a greying beard or whiskers, and Macassar oil to style their hair. The latter was made from a mixture of coconut oil, palm oil and ying ylang. According to the advertisements circulating at this time, Macassar oil did not just hold one's hair in place, it also encouraged growth and strengthened one's locks. The widespread use of hair oil among men brought about a change in home décor too. Women bought or made antimacassars, namely strips of linen to cover chair arms and headrests to prevent soiling of chairs and sofas when men came to visit and sat resting their heads (covered in hair oil) on the furniture.

Excessive use of cosmetics by the male members of society, that is, pretty much anything beyond the hair products, could prove seriously detrimental to their role in public life. Take the case of Martin Van Buren, for example, who looked like being the winner in the 1840 American presidential election year and lost because his rival Charles Ogle accused him of excessive and unnecessary personal spending; 'supplying his toilet with double extract of Queen Victoria ... eau de cologne ... Corinthian oil of cream ... of eglantine ... Mr Van Buren sees fit to spend his cash buying these and other perfumes and cosmetics for his toilet.' This is, I suppose, the nineteenth-century equivalent of Richard Nixon's 'five o'clock shadow', allegedly one of the reasons why he failed to secure the American presidency in 1960. It all came down to appearances.

Nature versus Artifice

Despite being fashionable, opinions remain divided as to whether or not cosmetics should, in fact, be worn at all. Both sides of the argument expressed their ideas in extremes. The Church continued to disapprove of make-up but the idea that wearing cosmetics was a form of deceit prevailed outside the realms of the Church too. According to the poet Longfellow (1807–1882), 'often treachery lies beneath the fairest hair'. For the opposite side of the debate note the views expressed in *The Art of Beauty or The Best Methods of Improving and Preserving the Shape Carriage and Complexion* (1825);

> Ought to people to use paint? Why not? When a person is young and fresh and handsome to paint would be perfectly ridiculous; it would be wantonly spoiling the fairest gifts of nature. But on the contrary, when an antique and veneral dowager covers her brown and shrivelled skin with a thick layer of white paint heightened with a tint of vermillion we are sincerely thankful to her for then we can look at her at least without disgust.

Consider too the satirical piece entitled *A Defense of Cosmetics* first published in 1894 by Max Beerbohm, later a newspaper magnate but at the time a Cambridge student with, it seems, time on his hands:

> The white cliffs of Albion shall be ground to powder for loveliness and perfumed by the ghost of many a little violet.
> The fluffy elder ducks that are swimming round the pond shall lose their feathers that the powder puff may be moon like as it passes over loveliness's face.

Nature itself (that is landscape and bird life) is destroyed for the sake of cosmetics. While this is certainly tongue in cheek, the idea that artifice could sound the death knell of nature was not new. The constant friction between the two ideologies, nature and artifice, had existed for centuries but despite all the debate that had gone before, in the nineteenth century the question of which one was superior to the other remained unresolved. To an extent whether, in reality, nature or artifice, that is to say, the unpainted or painted face was in vogue, was rather a fashion in its own right. The rhetorical argument meanwhile raged on.

The Dangers of Cosmetics

There were many dangers that were encountered and had to be overcome as a consequence of living in the nineteenth century. This was true no matter whether you were rich or poor. These hazards included the unhealthy London fog and the industrial smog that was regularly encountered in other cities too. There was also the threat of disease that, at that time, could not be simply cured, as well as the dangers of using machinery in an industrialised age when there was little or no protection in the workplace.

Cosmetics made from harmful ingredients were just another potential hazard. There were plenty of beauty products on the market that were harmful; for example, mercury was used as a bleaching agent in both hair and face products. It is clear that caution was still necessary when buying and using make-up. Women were warned to beware of misleading advertisements in the press, and of the perils of buying from travelling salesmen. One nineteenth-century periodical comments:

People should avoid the use of cosmetics the composition of which they are unacquainted. There are cosmetics which at first produce an astonishing effect and ultimately ruin the skin. Females should therefore abstain in general from all the cosmetics which are offered them by empirics.

Undoubtedly this was sound and sensible advice. In the absence of any regulation, the onus was on the individual to use products that could be trusted –or suffer the consequences. There was no legal comeback or financial refund for a dissatisfied, or even disfigured, customer and there were plenty of quacks and street sellers willing to sell their wares to those who believed their sales talk and promotions. *The Ladies Monthly Magazine* dated 1801 states:

> All contrivances of craft empirics perfumers travelling mountebanks &c ... which are pompously offered to the public in daily prints or by means of bills or pamphlets containing specious certificates to induce the giddy, the idle and unwary multitude (nay sometimes ladies of rank and fashion) to purchase those 'beautifying compositions' are mournful instances off human folly and moral depravity.

However, ladies of fashion were avid magazine readers for enjoyment, fascination, information and instruction, and despite such warnings, they might easily be tempted by extravagant claims and exotic-sounding products advertised in such publications. Thankfully, the same article, having condemned cosmetics then goes on to give recipes that the author does consider acceptable and which seem, from a modern standpoint, to be safe to use; for example, a cream made from honey and wheaten flour to soften and care for the hands and face. To condemn the use of make-up but go on to give details and recipes considered least noxious while always excluding the most dangerous was a common journalistic approach in nineteenth century books and magazines that gave instructions about make-up. After all, magazines depended to an extent for their revenue on advertisements and therefore it would not do to be seen to contradict their claims. Publications were inclined to adopt a similar line to the one taken in following example from *The Ladies Book of Useful Information* (1896):

'We do not approve of face washes but as some ladies will use them we recommend the following as harmless.' Problematically, contemporary writers on make-up did not always agree on what was and what was not safe to use. This particular text notes that dampening the face with glycerine tempered with rosewater then powder with the finest magnesia as safe, and goes on to record the purchase of five cents' worth of bismuth of flake white, as well as powder chalk mixed with of rosewater. The author does, however, add a note of caution in respect of the second mixture 'Great care must be taken to wash off this preparation before retiring to rest as bismuth is of a hurtful nature.' Glycerine could be dangerous too, depending on its source but no mention is made of that.

Once a product was purchased it might be down to the ladies' servants to test it in the home, for safety and authenticity. In the *Duties of a Lady's Maid* (1825) by J. Bulcock, the said servant is advised 'the makers of rouge out of economy sometimes substitute cinnabar for carmine. You should ascertain if the carmine be genuine which will be the case if it not altered whether by a mixture of salt or sorrel or by that of alkali'. Cinnabar was highly poisonous while the insect dye carmine was entirely safe for application.

Cost might be prohibitive when purchasing an unadulterated product. *The Ladies Book of Useful Information* anonymously published in 1896 recommends a skin preparation for the face and hands made from water distilled from a plant grown on the banks of the Volga River in Russia. Pure this might be but imagine the price such an unusual product sourced not only from a great distance but from an exotic sounding location might have fetched. The general populace could not have afforded such cosmetics, which often came with a significant price tag inflated by their pedigree. Some advocated avoidance of products with too many ingredients, or cheaper versions of a powder or face cream in which the main ingredient had been adulterated in some way; it was best to use pure talcum powder for example. The initial beneficial effects of some of the more dangerous cosmetics tempted the buyer. *Beauty culture* by H Ellen Browning (1898) explains the problem: 'Many of the toilet preparations sold for this purpose contain bismuth, or other ingredients of a similar kind, which affect their purpose very rapidly, but do not help in preserving beauty of complexion, because they are injurious to the skin in the long run.'

Women's Magazines

By the middle of the nineteenth century there were no less than 100 magazines for women in publication across Europe. Some took a firm stance against the use of make-up. For example, *The Leisure Hour Magazine* published in 1867 discouraged the lightening of hair. However, as this was a magazine published by a religious organisation its stated opposition to make-up is hardly surprising. *Vogue* began publication in 1892 and in its first year this magazine also struck a note of caution, advising that a 'cosmetic which at first produces an astonishing effect can ultimately ruin the skin'. Other magazines, however, wholeheartedly embraced the subject carrying regular news, advertisements and advice about make-up. *Harpers Bazaar* had a regular column written by their resident beauty expert, and known as *The Ugly Girl Papers*. By popular demand these articles were compiled into an anthology. Aside from carrying advertisements to persuade women to purchase various products, they contained plenty of recipes for making make-up at home. Here is an example taken from *The Ugly Girl Papers,* which offers what the writer describes as a 'harmless' and 'cheap' and indeed 'elegant' preparation for whitening the face and neck ... 'made from terebinth of Mecca three grains ; oil of sweet almonds four ounces, spermaceti two drachms, flour of zinc one drachm; white wax two drachms; rose water six drachms'. The method of preparation was simple; basically mix with warm water to melt. All of the ingredients would have been readily available for purchase at the chemist's shop. An American monthly magazine entitled *Godey's Ladies Book* began circulation in 1830, established by Louis Antoine Godey with the purpose of educating American women. Certainly over the years the magazine carried accomplished writing by such famous authors as Edgar Allan Poe and Harriet Beecher Stowe but the readers themselves were often the contributors, showing themselves interested in discussing make-up as well as fashions in dress. The magazine combined not only literary essays but also advice on how to care for your teeth, how to make a toilet water and look after one's complexion alongside recipes for apple pudding and other wholesome cooking. The cookery and the make-up are very much in the tradition of the eighteenth century books for women but the quality stories and essays show the female readership of the magazine, and others like it, to be educated and at the same time interested in their looks.

Make-up and the Stage

Actresses wore make-up, often to excess, both off as well as on the stage. In the theatre the actors were under considerable scrutiny, by the very nature of the event, especially from the audience sitting close to the stage. If they appeared unsuitable, perhaps too old or ugly for the part they were playing, then the performer might find herself (or indeed himself) out of work and in poverty. Concealing the signs of old age was a necessity for women in particular if they were to keep working and earning money at the top of their profession. Their appearance in public was often an extension of their on-stage life. The renowned actress Mary Robinson was spotted in James Street off Pall Mall by the diarist and gossip Laetitia Hawkins (1759–1835) 'perhaps dressed as the belle of Hyde Park trimmed powdered patched painted to the utmost powder of rouge and white lead'. Portraits of actresses were very popular towards the middle to end of the nineteenth century. The term double embellishment was used to describe paintings of famous actresses where they are painted in the normal sense but then heavily made-up on top of that; the portrait by Thomas Gainsborough of dancer Giovanna Baccelli is one good example.

Greasepaint, or make-up composed of a coloured pigment mixed with lard for the stage, was invented in Germany in the 1850s. Leichner was one of the main cosmetic manufactures that produced make-up for the stage in the nineteenth century, but well-known actresses including Lillie Langtry and Sarah Bernhardt endorsed specific brands of make-up for everyday use by women in general. Lillie Langtry promoted the 'harmless' Pears Soap (which was and is indeed harmless) while Sarah Bernhardt advertised an equally benign product with the fancy French name *la Diaphane Poudre De Riz*; this was, in effect, rice powder. Although celebrated actresses wore make-up extensively both on stage and off, better class ladies were not expected to follow their example. However, these actresses were the women who had the attention of eminent men, in their roles as mistresses and confidantes, therefore there was some pressure on the wives of these male philanderers who associated with actresses to copy and compete with them.

Hair

In the nineteenth century there was a move away from frequenting the barbershop. These premises had a acquired an unfavourable reputation as being too popular with men until the late hours of the night and had in some cases become little more than drinking dens. The first public hair salons exclusively for women opened in 1800. Bond street hairdressers Robert Douglas and rival H. P. Trueffitt even hired women to work for them. The original impetus for employing women came as a result of their male assistants going on strike. These employers found women were cheaper to hire. Not only was the wage bill smaller (of course the notion of equal pay for men and women did not exist) but hiring women as hairdressers offered the opportunity to attract a different clientele;

that is, middle-class women and society ladies. Salons sometimes catered for the male customer too but where this was the case, men and women called at these premises via separate entrances so neither should suffer the embarrassment of catching one another needing their hair done or indeed in the process of having their hair attended to and therefore in any sort of disarray. In a hairdresser's shop the female client had her hair washed, face forward, and styled, rather than cut. Women did not regularly cut their hair unless they became ill. When someone is described as having their hair dressed or done, this was more about having it styled. A sprinkling of rosewater on the hair to finish might be offered as part of the service and as an extra luxurious touch. Hairdressing salons also sold manufactured goods such as Rowland's Macassar oil used by men to keep their hair in place.

Hair powder had acted as a sort of dry shampoo and with its demise, one's hair needed to be washed more often. Women may have been looking for something more effective to wash their hair. Shampoo was an Indian word that originally meant having a massage. Shampoo as we know it did not become commercially available until the early twentieth century when a product that we would recognise as shampoo was invented by Kasey Herbert; however, the Berlin chemist Hans Schwarzkopf did invent a sort of powdered product for washing hair in 1898. In the nineteenth century, a concoction to condition the hair made of stinging nettles was popular and quite effective. Indeed nettles are rich in minerals and plant hormones and valued today in shampoos and conditioners for these properties, which can encourage hair growth and promote shine.

There were plenty of dangerous concoctions, though thankfully also safer alternatives, that could be used at home to keep one's hair clean as an excerpt from the magazine *The Young Ladies' Journal* (1873) points out: 'washing your hair with soda will make it lighter: but it is injurious to the skin of the head and causes the hair to break. Rosemary is very beneficial and is used as a wash'. The latter is still used in hair tonics today. Another safe example of homemade hair care using readily available household ingredients comes from the earlier publication *The Mirror of Graces* written by, quote, 'a Lady of Distinction' in 1811:

> This is a cleanser and brightener of the head and hair, and should be applied in the morning. Beat up the whites of six eggs into froth, and with that anoint the head close to the roots of the hair. Leave it to dry on; Then wash the head and hair thoroughly with a mixture of rum and rosewater in equal quantities.

Hair Dyes

Where blonde hair had always been in vogue, fashion now enthusiastically embraced the brunette too. In 1854, the songwriter Stephen Foster wrote his popular lyric, 'I dream of Jeanie with the light brown hair'. According to Cooley's *Instructions and Cautions Respecting the Selection and the Use of Perfumes, Cosmetics and other Toilet Articles* published in 1873, to darken her hair or to cover grey a lady might use a lead comb. Caution or rather abstention would have been the better choice here. A recipe book entitled somewhat unimaginatively *Six Hundred Valuable Receipts* (1860) recommends the frugal use of alkanet root, scented, tied up and stored in bags. There was skill required in matching the hair colour with one's complexion as *Beauty Culture* (1898) acknowledges: 'Indeed, dyeing the hair almost necessitates making up the complexion, too, and unless both these operations are most skilfully performed they fail to express their raison d'être, being inartistic, and therefore not beautiful'. Women, as ever, had to deal with unwanted hair too. A pitch plaster or a piece of leather made duly sticky with gum or resin was applied to remove any unsightly body hair.

Wigs and Hairpieces

A lady or gentleman might wish to purchase a hair piece. These became briefly popular after 1855, until around 1868, when they became less fashionable. Chignons were exported in large numbers from France to Britain. In the mid-century, French and Italian hair was particularly coveted and surprisingly, perhaps both from a modern perspective and if we look back in history too, grey and white hair was the most expensive. This despite the fact that youthful looks were at a premium not only as a bargaining chip in the marriage market but also in the nineteenth century in the labour market. Grey or white hair had previously been associated with unattractive aging and, to an extent, this is still the case today. When not the height of fashion, hair-pieces were still worn but discreetly advertised, as 'imperceptible hair coverings'. Full wigs too became discreet, not least because there was a belief that women who were bald were descended from sufferers of syphilis, otherwise known as The French Pox. Baldness among women was certainly not desirable but the obvious wearing of full wigs so popular in the previous century was no longer considered tasteful or *a la mode*. A woman obviously wearing a wig was thought to intend trickery or deceit. Nevertheless the continued use of lead-based make-up as well as illness would have resulted in hair loss and so sometimes necessitated false hair. Wigs were no longer fashionable for men either. Men wearing wigs were regarded as vain. In effect, whether man or woman, only one's hairdresser should know if their client was wearing a wig.

Skin Care

To meet the standards of beauty of the day, all exposed skin should resemble porcelain – white and unblemished. Men might still judge a lady's beauty by her hands. According to *The Lady's Guide to Perfect Gentility* (1856), 'an elegant hand is regarded by many as betokening evident prestige in its possessor. Indeed some persons especially gentleman make the hand a test of beauty calling a lady pretty however ugly she may be otherwise if she only can display a beautiful hand.' The author goes on to recommend a paste made from a mixture of sweet almonds, breadcrumbs, spring water, brandy and eggs for this purpose. The fashion for low-cut dresses meant attention needed to be paid not only to the face and hands, but also to the arms, shoulders but also to the décolletage. There was a mid-Victorian trend for drawing blue veins onto pale skin as a mark of beauty and status, a practice for which there was a precedent in the fifteenth and sixteenth centuries.

A fair complexion remained the hallmark of gentility and status. *The Lady's Guide to Perfect Gentility* recommended using lemon juice mixed with sugar candy and leaf gold to achieve a fair complexion. This recipe uses the lemon itself as the receptacle with the rind removed and the lemon roasted in hot ashes. The inclusion of the gold would make what was otherwise an inexpensive product beyond the purse of the average woman of the time. Anything made from roses was popular, and probably beneficial. According to a September edition of the periodical *The London Pioneer* (1847) English milk of roses consisted of one pint of rosewater, one pound of subcarbonate of potass [potash] and half-a-pint of olive oil. To make French milk of roses according to the same article, one needed to add a few extra ingredients namely, 'sixty drops of lavender oil and three of otto [attar] of roses' The instructions given read, 'dissolve in a quarter of a pint of spirits of wine'. The latter mixture is more sophisticated, heavily scented and no doubt more expensive.

Freckles were still regarded as unwanted blemishes, though they had largely lost their association with witchcraft and devilry. The favourite cosmetic for removing freckles in trendsetting Paris consisted of an ounce of alum and an ounce of lemon juice blended in a pint of rosewater. Beauty masks containing natural ingredients such as honey, eggs, milk, oatmeal as well as juice of fruits and vegetables were popular and could be effective in clearing the face and freshening the complexion. Plumpers were still in use. Alex Ross, the inventor of a machine to correct a crooked nose, sold these as a means of correcting the shape of the face. His advertisement in *The London Daily News* in 1891 states that 'plumpers for thin faces are placed in the mouth between the teeth and the cheeks making the profile perfect and the shape of the face correct. They are the colour of the gums and easy to wear'. His plumpers were available by post for 21s. Ponds Cold Cream was first produced in 1846 and was basically a trademarked modern version of Galen's original cold cream from Roman times. Mineral Oil Cold Cream, also called Perfect Cold Cream, was marketed from 1890. Lanolin, the natural grease extracted from sheep's wool, which had also been used as in skin care in the Roman period, was reintroduced in 1882 by the company Brown & Leibreich. The American publication *Godey's Lady's Book* suggests brown butcher's paper soaked in apple vinegar, an application reminiscent of the old nursery rhyme Jack and Jill in which Jack finishes up with his head wrapped in vinegar and brown paper, intended, in his case, to draw out any bruises; this would probably have exfoliated and softened skin as well.

Face Powders

Face powders could be bought cheaply in unmarked packets from chemists' shops, where they were either made up on the premises or bought in wholesale. These inexpensive cosmetics were often made from potato, rice or maize starch, scented with orris root. The chemist John Scoffern writing this time in *The Belgravia Magazine* in 1868 notes that,

> Pearl powders, which are a popular modern cosmetic, are variously made. Some are nothing else than powdered talc or French chalk; others a mixture of the same with common

chalk; a third order contains starch grains mingled with the preceding one, or both. By starch grains I meant to signify the preparation known as 'violet powder', which really has no more to do with violets than it has with cabbages or cucumbers.

Orris root, and not violet powder, was often used as a scent. If a lady wished to purchase a more sophisticated product in fancy packaging then the price, of course, went up. As ever the inclusion of a scent from France, or even a French name, hiked the price. Take for example *Duvet de Ninon*, advertised as follows:

> One of the most agreeable cosmetics is rice powder but it needs to be chosen with care for many face powders are unhealthy or dangerous. The best of all is Duvet de Ninon the finest and most adhesive and impalpable known it is eminently hygienic and gives the skin a dazzling whiteness.

Duvet de Ninon is supplied by the Perfumerie Ninon, 31 Rue de Quatre Septembre, Paris.

In 1897 some analysis of face powders was undertaken following concerns raised about the content of the more expensive products at a conference of hairdressers in Paris. The results obtained from the examination of eight different powders were subsequently published in the edition of *The British Medical Journal* for that year. Though they came to no conclusive decision, these eminent hairdressers did advise caution, having found that while some of the face powders might simply be made from rice powder, others contained dangerous metals such as lead, bismuth and zinc. Using bismuth could result in skin paralysis. This metal also turned black if near a fire giving quite the opposite effect of the bleached whites it was intended to achieve.

A book entitled *Beauty its Attainment and Preservation* first published in 1892 gives a detailed description of the popular technique known as enamelling, favoured by eminent women including Princess Alexandra, the wife of King Edward VII.

In enamelling the face the skin is first prepared by an alkaline wash after which all wrinkles and depressions are filled with a yielding paste. The face is simply painted and artists in this time generally prefer to use the poisonous salts of lead for the purpose as they produce more striking effects than any other pigment. After the white layer is applied the red tinting is done.

Enamelling led to an awkward and curious problem, which could have far-reaching implications. A lady's face was in effect rendered frozen and immobile by this process, making communication with others difficult. Women found it difficult to adopt different facial expressions (such as smiling or frowning) without spoiling their make-up. No doubt, on occasion, this lack of ability to express one's true feelings had the potential to result in a deal of confusion. Nevertheless this was all the rage among society ladies, especially as it had royal approval in the shape of Princess Alix no less.

According to Browning, in her work *Beauty Culture* (1898): 'Wrinkles are the result of pouting, frowning, making a martyr of oneself, meeting troubles half-way, and looking on the blackest side of things.' The author follows her explanation for the causes of wrinkles with a recipe for wrinkle lotion, 'to be painted on thrice daily consisting of the following ingredients with proportions; one and a half ounces of tannin, seven ounces of rose water, three ounces of glycerine, and half an ounce of Eau de Cologne'. Another recipe, and a somewhat cheaper alternative, could be made up from one ounce of lemon juice, one ounce of eau de cologne, one ounce of simple tincture of benzoin and two ounces of distilled water. Paraffin was even used as cosmetic filler for deep wrinkles.

Apart from applying creams, powders or lotions to one's face there were other methods that could cultivate the desired pale complexion and prevent signs of aging. Some were practical, while others were more dangerous. One practical step was to invest in heavy curtains in your home to protect the female occupants from the sun and to be certain to carry a parasol if going outside. A more dangerous option was to ingest something that might induce a pale complexion. Women drank vinegar to this end. Vinegar was rumoured to have been a factor in the death of Lizzie Siddall, the famous red-haired muse of the Pre-Raphaelite poet and painter Dante Rossetti. However, it is equally likely that she had naturally pale skin, a common feature among people with red hair.

Rouge

According to Susan Sibbald (1763–1866), the wife of a Scottish laird who wrote her memoirs late in life, 'to rouge highly was then all the rage and without your cheeks the colour of a peony you were not *a la mode*'. Rouge could be made from red sandalwood, cochineal, brazilwood or saffron mixed with talcum powder. The red and yellow flowers of the herb safflower also made popular powdered rouge. Liquid rouge was known as bloom. Some rouge such as carmine made from cochineal produced a very brilliant red, which was sometimes toned down by the addition of hair powder for a more subtle effect. The intention, at this time, was to create a natural looking blush. Cinnabar or red lead was still in use despite being known to be highly dangerous, but the mineral dye red ochre was safe and had, of course, been used since prehistoric times. Rouge could be purchased from various outlets such as pharmacies or perfumers and, in the later years of the nineteenth century, department stores. It was sold in pots, glass jars or a book of papers impregnated with colour and was applied using one's fingers, cotton wool, a brush or even a hare's foot. *The New Family Receipt Book* (1811) gives the following recipe for rouge; 'take carmine in fine powder one part and levigated French chalk five parts, mix'. French chalk is unscented talcum powder, also used by tailors to mark out patterns, by dry cleaners today to remove greasy marks from fabric, and in joiner's workshops as a lubricant. In 1863 the cosmetic company Bourjois manufactured the first compact rouge made simply from baking powder with colorant added. There were even instructions available on how to make some commercially produced products to try at home. *Harpers Bazaar* in its regular column *The Ugly Girl Papers* (1875) gives a recipe for Devoux French Rouge consisting of: 'Carmine half a drachm, oil of almonds one drachm, French chalk two ounces. Mix'. This makes dry rouge. Multi-use products also existed. Smith's Rosebud Salve (1895) an American product promised kissable lips, but could also be used to tame flyaway hair, as a rouge, as an eyebrow groomer and was even recommended for cuts and grazes. Its pretty packaging was also a selling point. A lady in haste might still resort to a dampened red ribbon. As dyes were not fast, she need only rub her cheeks with the ribbon for the colour to come off on her cheeks and affect a hint of rouge.

Lips, Teeth and Eyes

At the very beginning of the century, salves to keep lips moist were popular. *The New Family Recipe Book* (1811) includes the following recipe for a red lip salve;

Take a pound of olive oil and two ounces of root alkanet, macerate with heat until the oil is well coloured then add two ounces of spermaceti (whale blubber) eight ounces of white wax and twelve ounces of suet. When nearly cold stir in a drachm of orange flower water and 1 half drachm of lavender.

This is a very greasy mixture, made at home in a large batch to be stored for some considerable period of time for use perhaps by the whole family, as the title of the book in which this appears would suggest.

Six Hundred Valuable Receipts, which includes recipes not only for cosmetics and medicines but also for the treatment for horses and advice on making of wines and spirits, prescribes the following lip-salve,

> take two ounces oil of lemon, one ounce white wax. one ounce spermaceti. Melt these ingredients, and while warm add two ounces of rose-water, and one ounce of orange-flower water. These make Hudson's cold cream,—a very excellent article. The lips are liable to excoriation and chaps, which often extend to considerable depth. These chaps are generally occasioned by mere cold.

Glycerine, which was safe when it was sold as a by-product of the candle making industry and not sourced from the processing of lead plaster, served as a lip salve as well as a skin cream and hair oil. Lip salves were used not for vanity but for protection. However, in 1880, Guerlain, a family firm established in 1828, manufactured the first commercially produced lipstick made of grapefruit butter and wax with a hint of natural colour. This innovative rose-tinted product was sold in a tube and given the name Forget-me-not.

Not only lips but teeth should be in good order, if for no other reason than to avoid gum disease and bad breath. Sir Washington Sheffield, an eminent London dentist, began selling toothpaste in a tube in 1892. The *Lady's Guide to Perfect Gentility* recommends drops of hydrochloric acid mixed with lemon juice and sugar to counteract bad breath, a mixture, on account of the inclusion of hydrochloric acid, that is, effectively, bleach; this was more likely to corrode one's innards than cure halitosis. Even breathing in the fumes might cause one to choke. Other safer tooth preparations contained chalk, animal bone, myrrh (a natural analgesic) and even charcoal.

To make their eyelashes and eyebrows look darker and more obvious, women continued to use the juice of elderberries, burnt cork or cloves – though wealthier ladies might apply a black made from frankincense and mastic. This mixture, it was claimed, did not come off with perspiration; the added feature perhaps justified the extra expense. The dilating effect on one's pupils of using belladonna added to the consumptive look considered attractive at this time; its use continued, despite the potentially severe side effects. The cosmetic company Rimmel produced the first mascara made of coal dust and petroleum jelly.

Shopping

The mechanisation brought about by the Industrial Revolution allowed companies to produce make-up on a large scale although some products, such as face creams, still had a limited shelf life. Shop bought goods became widely available. Make-up of all sorts could be purchased in the early part of the nineteenth century from pharmacies and perfumers. In 1817 there were five perfume sellers in Oxford Street, London, alone. At the Great Exhibition of 1851, a wide and attractive range of beauty products were on show. Some were exhibited before the public in ostentatious manner; Rimmel advertised their wares with a perfume fountain that drew much attention. In all, there were 727 exhibitors in the spa and perfume section, including Knight, Gibbs and Yardley. They all gave away free samples to advertise their products. However, a ticket to the exhibition itself was not cheap. A season ticket for gentleman cost £3 3s while the charge was £2 2s for ladies. Over the days, the price did drop but the cost of entry and the products themselves were not within the price range of the poorer classes. Many of the companies that exhibited are familiar names to us today, Guerlain, Bourjois, Cyclax and Gibbs for example. Generally these companies had entered the market selling one or maybe two specific products. For example, Bourjois originally sold rouge. Colgate started selling toothpaste powder, or paste in cake form, in 1873 – but the year before the company began by selling its Cashmere Bouquet soap.

The first department store, Le Bon Marche, opened its doors in Paris in 1852. In London, Selfridges opened its make-up counter in the 1890s. In Emile Zola's novel *The Ladies' Paradise*, first published in 1883, the author describes the department store in which much of his story takes place in lavish detail:

> Inside the display counters and on the small crystal shelves of the showcases pomades and creams were lined up boxes of powder and rouge phials of oils and toilet waters ... the customers were delighted by a silver fountain in the centre a shepherdess standing in a harvest of flowers from which a continuous trickle of violet water was flowing tinkling musically in the medal basin. An exquisite scent was spreading everywhere and the ladies soaked their handkerchiefs in it as they passed.

The department store was, in effect, a more permanent form of the temporary Great Exhibition of 1851, which had so excited the public. Although this is fiction, it recalls for example the famous scented fountain erected by Rimmel at the Great Exhibition.

The Victorian novelist Charlotte Yonge (1823–1901) was widely read and admired during her lifetime, although her novels are no longer in print. In her description of the shop owned by her character Cora Darke in her novel *Love and Life* (1880) Yonge gives us an idea of what a smaller shop premises might have been like in the Victorian period, both exotic and exciting, stocked with every cosmetic imaginable. We get a sense of the smells and the thrills that awaited the women who entered such premises,

> ...a little cupboard of a room, scented with as compound of every imaginable perfume. Bottles of every sort of essence pomade and cosmetics were ranged on the shelves, or within glass doors. Interspersed with masks, boxes for patches, bunches of false hair, powder puffs, curling irons, rare feathers. An alembic was in the fireplace and pen and ink in a strangely shaped Standish were on the table.

Of course not every fashionable lady or indeed gentleman lived in the big cities. As a result, mail order was a popular means by which the women and men, especially those who lived in the great houses outside the cities could purchase the beauty products they desired. Trent's depilatory or hair remover was one product available by post for the price of one pound. Duvet de Ninon, that popular face powder, was initially only available to order by post from Paris. Avon, founded in 1886 by a travelling salesman named David McConnell, provided another means of purchase and sale; door-to-door sales were, effectively, a rather more regular and organised version of the travelling pedlar.

American Influence
Products manufactured in the United States flooded into Europe. Wealthy heiresses, who belonged to prestigious American families, sought high-status marriages with titled gentlemen, particularly those who were destined to inherit the family fortune and a stately home. These women, who became known as the Dollar Princesses, brought fashion and style with them. That included their make-up. Gloria Vanderbilt, Duchess of Marlborough and first wife of Charles Spencer-Churchill, is one notable example. The Americans brought with them their own manufactured idea of feminine

beauty too. Known as the Gibson Girl she was not in fact one single person at all, instead the painter Charles Dana Gibson drew his inspiration for her portrait from a concoction of American women who modelled for him in the 1890s. Stage actress Camille Clifford was just one of these women. The Gibson Girl represented perfection in female beauty. Among her many attributes was soft hair and that ever-coveted flawless pale complexion. Her eyes and lips were painted with natural colours, the fashion of the day. Her pale complexion still, as it always had done, represented wealth and status and the avoidance of demeaning manual labour.

Madame Recamier was the trade name of a successful American cosmetics business owned and run by Harriet Hubbard Ayer. The eponymous madame was a famous beauty from Napoleonic times, so Harriet deemed this a suitable name for her company. Harriet Hubbard Ayer claimed 'women under thirty need no cosmetics' and was hence known especially for her quality face creams and anti-aging products, which we assume she intended for use by older women. Recamier wrinkle treatment, for example, was billed as 'the successful tissue builder'. However Harriet's company manufactured other products for use by society in general. These included a lotion for 'removing dust from the face after travelling'. The same product is also described 'as invaluable to gentlemen to be used after shaving'. Advertisements for her products claimed that they were endorsed and used 'by the most beautiful women of every century'; of course, this was impossible as the products had not been available in previous centuries but this is did not matter as there was no legal comeback.

Cosmetics in Court

On account of their value, cosmetics were worth stealing. Also being often relatively small in size, a lipstick, small bottle of lotion or a tin of powder might be easily pocketed and sold for a profit. Harsh penalties were meted out in the nineteenth century for those apprehended and charged even with what we would consider minor crimes. Therefore a thief caught stealing a lipstick or powder was likely to be subject to a heavy penalty. In 1809, according to the records of the Old Bailey, London's central criminal court, one Brunswick Bailey aged thirteen was imprisoned for three months for stealing 'one bottle of oil value 8*d*: one bottle of paint 1*s* six grains of rouge 4*d* nine grains of carmine 6*d*'. The items are described as the property of his master, Samuel Crouch, most likely purchased by him for his wife to use.

Cosmetics, Murder and Madeleine Smith

Cosmetics played their part in much more serious illegal activity too. The case of Madeleine Smith versus the Crown caused a considerable amount of scandal, not only on account of the seriousness of the crime (murder) but also because of the lurid details described in court, the length of the trial and the final verdict. The details of the case were widely covered in the press. Tales of murder were the very fodder of cheap nineteenth century magazines and newspapers whose readership lapped up every detail. Madeleine Smith, a twenty-two-year-old woman and a member of the Scottish aristocracy, was accused of having murdered her secret lover, Emile L'Angelier, a lowly gardener. He was found dead on 23 March 1857 with eighty-eight grains of arsenic in his stomach. Madeleine was arrested and charged with his murder eight days later. Tried in her home city of Glasgow, Madeleine Smith admitted to having purchased arsenic but stated, in the words of *The Illustrated London News* (1857), that 'she used [this] in washing, as a cosmetic'. The court controversially handed down a verdict of 'not proven', a judgement allowed in Scots Law when there was not enough evidence to convict or acquit.

Arsenic was cheap and readily available. On a shopping list its presence would not raise eyebrows as it had many legitimate uses at this time, including as a cosmetic. Robert Dick in *The Connection of Health and Beauty or the Dependence of a Pleasing Face and Figure on Physical Intellectual and Moral Regulation* published in 1857 even records the supposed benefits of arsenic to the complexion:

> It is said that by dose of a quarter of a grain gradually increased to the large amount of ten grains daily, a trebly fatal dose to persons not gradually inured to it, a pale thin woman with few or no suitors is often metamorphosed into a well conditioned blooming creature with glowing cheeks and sparkling eyes and as natural and intended consequence a band of young admirers of the opposite sex.

A young woman needed marriage to a husband who could support her. Using cosmetics wasn't merely a matter of aesthetics but of survival and even if there were known dangers, these were often seen as worth the risk. Whether Madeleine Smith was guilty of murder or not, she saw fit to leave Scotland, remarry abroad and start a new life.

Florence Maybrick and the Case of the Cosmetic Flypapers

Florence Maybrick was tried for the murder of her husband James Maybrick in 1889. As a young woman travelling from America she had met and married James Maybrick, who was many years her senior. Their relationship hit the rocks when James, a travelling salesman, carried on affairs and ran up debts. Florence, for her part, grew bored and fractious. James worried about his health like many people of the time and took a number of poisonous concoctions, including arsenic which was believed, in small doses, to be beneficial. Florence was alleged to have taken advantage of his hypochondriac tendencies and was brought to trial accused of soaking fly papers to extract the arsenic from them and using this poison to murder her husband. In her defence, Mrs Maybrick claimed that 'the fly papers were bought with the intention of using as a cosmetic'. She claimed to have been in the process of making a face wash prescribed for her by an American doctor in Brooklyn consisting of, among other things, arsenic, tincture of benzoin, and elderflower water. Florence narrowly escaped the gallows and after languishing in prison for fifteen years, died destitute in America. By a peculiar twist of fate, her deceased husband James Maybrick was later cited as a possible (even likely, given that the record of his movements indicate he was in the right places at the right times) fit for the notorious and savage murderer who terrorised London, namely Jack the Ripper.

Cosmetics and the Con Artist: The Infamous Madame Rachel

> Beautiful women –Madame Rachel begs to inform her lady patronesses the nobility and aristocracy generally that she has opened her annual subscription list for the supply of her costly Arabian reoperations for the restoration and preservation of female loveliness' which have obtained the patronage of royalty'.

This advertisement appeared in *The Morning Post* in March 1859. The text is peppered with words and promises to convince the wealthy that they not only wanted but needed to be a client of Madame Rachel's whose real name was Sarah Leverson. An opportunist of dubious character and from a humble background, Madame Rachel ran her business selling alleged oriental make-up in Bond Street, London. The products are described as costly and exotic, which added to their allure. Madame Rachel goes on in her advert to advise that these preparations are available only from her salon in new Bond Street. She had no other outlets. The middle man has been eliminated and the con woman got the entire proceeds from this obsequiously worded deception. Leverson preyed upon women's intrinsic fears about growing old. Despite the arrival of the department store and the option of buying cosmetics from perfumers' shops, wealthy women still called discreetly at premises like hers to be beautified. Madame Rachel and Mrs Frances Hemming (the latter owned and ran the House of Cyclax) offered anonymity to women who entered secretly, veiled, and hurried to private cubicles in their establishments. Their society acquaintances, indeed not even their friends, would not witness the lengths to which they would go and the expense they would incur in the name of beauty.

Although the prices of her product with their exotic names like Armenian liquid, Arab bloom powder, Alabaster liquid, Sultan's Beauty Wash or Magnetic Roc Dew Water of Sahara may not have been too excessive, when compared with others on the market at the time, Madame Rachel's fees for a course of treatment were hefty and women who became hooked on these and returned again and again to her premises ran up massive bills. Madame Rachel had no scruples when it came to taking women to court for non-payment of their accounts. These were accounts that their husbands often had no knowledge of, despite the fact men were legally bound at the time to settle any debts on behalf of their wives. At the old Bailey trial Cecelia Pearse versus Sarah Leverson, the amount of the bill accrued by Cecelia as payment for the cosmetic treatment of enamelling was considerable; 'thousand guineas and the process (that of enamelling) would take some months'. Repeated scandals over monies due to Madame Rachel resulted in changes in the law, making women more responsible for their own transactions and accounts.

The temptation to run up debt on cosmetics did nothing to assuage the male idea that women could not make rational

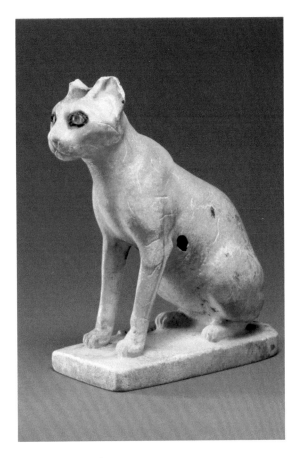

Right: Egyptian cosmetic vessel in the shape of a cat, *c*. 1990 BC. This is the earliest known three-dimensional representation of a cat in Egyptian art. (Courtesy of the Metropolitan Museum of Art, Purchase, Lila Acheson Wallace Gift, 1990)

Below: An Egyptian cosmetic box; because it is so plain it has proved difficult to date accurately, *c*. 1981–1550 BC. (Courtesy of the Metropolitan Museum of Art)

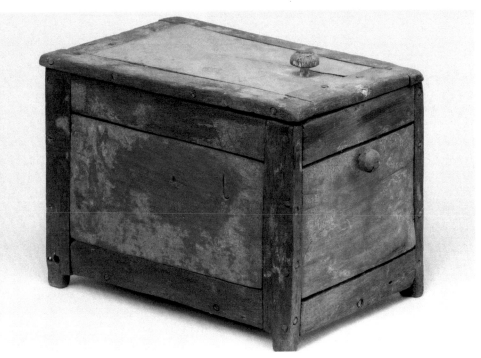

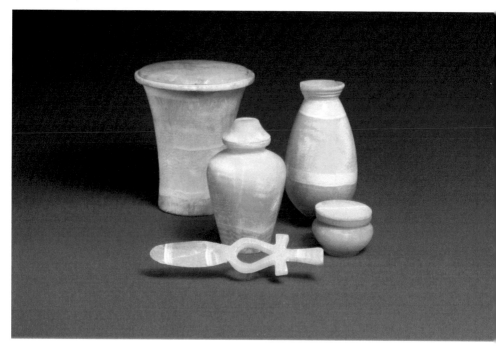

A group of stone cosmetic vessels from a tomb at Haraga, Egypt, *c.* 1887–1750 BC.
(Courtesy of the Metropolitan Museum of Art, Lila Acheson Wallace Gift, 2014)

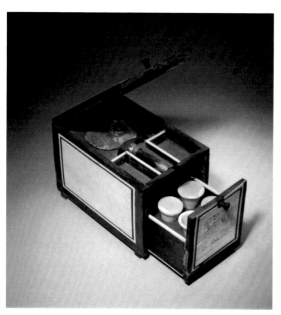
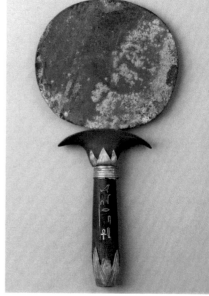

Above left: Cosmetic box of Kemeni and mirror of Reniseneb, *c.* 1814–1805 BC. The
box belonged to the royal butler Kemeni, who is depicted on one end making offerings to
the deified king Amenemhat IV. (Courtesy of the Metropolitan Museum of Art, Purchase,
Edward S. Harkness Gift, 1926)

Above right: Mirror of the chief of the southern Tens, Reniseneb, Egypt, *c.* 1810–1700 BC.
(Courtesy of the Metropolitan Museum of Art, Purchase, Edward S. Harkness Gift, 1926)

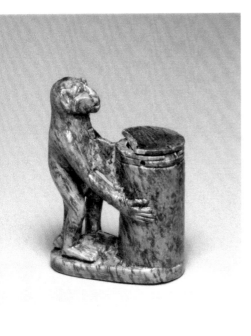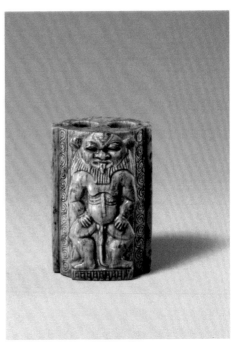

Above left: Egyptian kohl tube in the shape of a monkey holding a vessel, *c*. 1550–1450 BC. (Courtesy of the Metropolitan Museum of Art, Gift of Norbert Schimmel Trust, 1989)

Above right: Egyptian Kohl container decorated with Bes images, *c*. 1400 BC. (Courtesy of the Metropolitan Museum of Art, Purchase, Edward S. Harkness Gift, 1926)

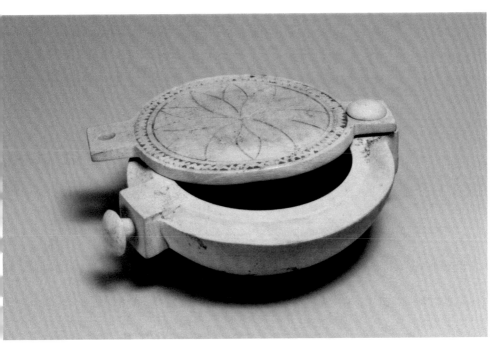

Egyptian cosmetic box with a swivel top, *c*. 1550–1458 BC. (Courtesy of the Metropolitan Museum of Art, Rogers Fund, 1916)

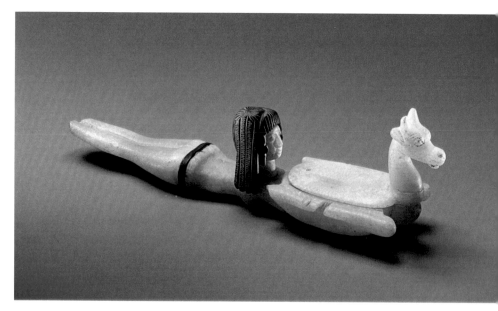

Cosmetic spoon in the shape of swimming woman holding a dish, *c.* 1390–1352 BC, reign of Amenhotep III. (Courtesy of the Metropolitan Museum of Art, Rogers Fund, 1926)

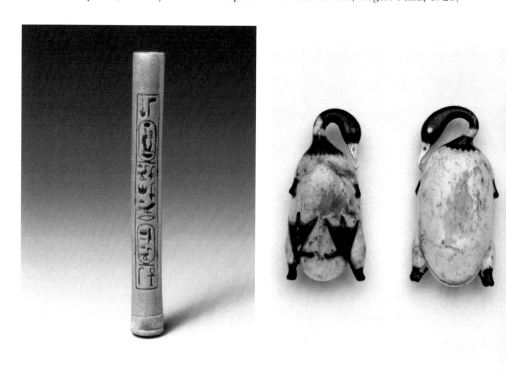

Above left: Egyptian Kohl tube inscribed for Amenhotep III and Princess Sitamun, *c.* 1390–1352 BC. (Courtesy of the Metropolitan Museum of Art, Purchase, Edward S. Harkness Gift, 1926)

Above right: Egyptian cosmetic dish in the shape of a trussed duck, *c.* 1353–1327 BC. (Courtesy of the Metropolitan Museum of Art, Rogers Fund, 1940)

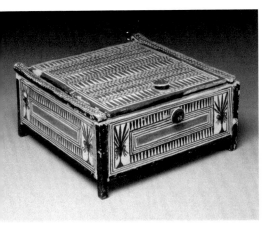 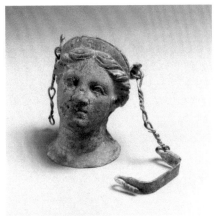

Above left: Decorated Egyptian cosmetic box from the tomb of Sennedjem, *c.* 1279–1213 BC. This one looks almost Art Deco. (Courtesy of the Metropolitan Museum of Art)

Above right: Etruscan Bronze balsamarium (cosmetics container), late fourth or early third century BC. Possibly depicting the goddess Turan or Lasa, patroness of lovers. (Courtesy of the Metropolitan Museum of Art, Rogers Fund, 1911)

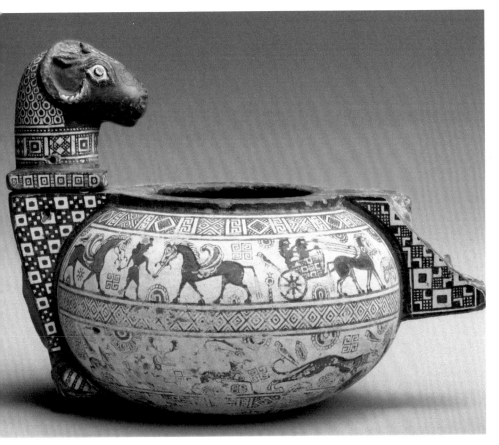

Terracotta cosmetic vase. Late sixth century BC. Eastern Greek. (Courtesy of the Metropolitan Museum of Art, The Bothmer Purchase Fund, 1977)

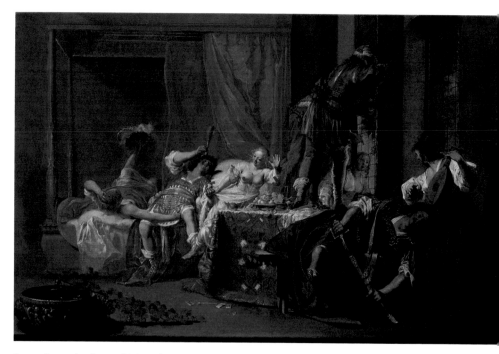

Scene from the lives of Messalina – a Roman example of the 'painted Jezebel' – and Gaius Silius, by Nicolaes Knüpfer, c. 1645–55. (Courtesy of the Rijksmuseum)

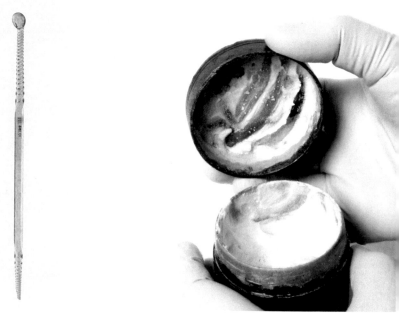

Above left: Glass ear pick, Roman, first century AD or later. (Courtesy of the Metropolitan Museum of Art, Gift of J. Pierpont Morgan, 1917)

Above right: The Londinium Cream, a canister containing cream from the Tabard Square Site, London, dated to the second century AD. (By kind permission of Pre-construct Archaeology Limited and the Museum of London)

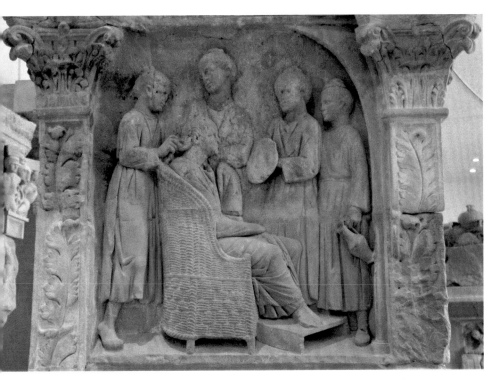

Funerary relief sculpture from Neumagen, Germany, third century AD, showing a woman at her toilet. (Rheinisches Landesmuseum, Trier)

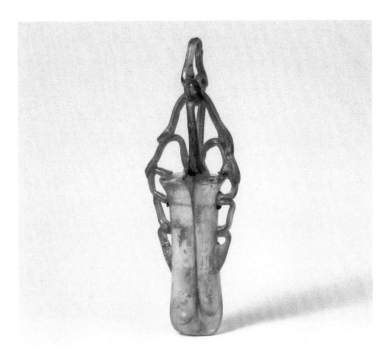

Glass double cosmetic flask (kohl tube), fourth or fifth century AD or later. Roman or Syrian. (Courtesy of the Metropolitan Museum of Art)

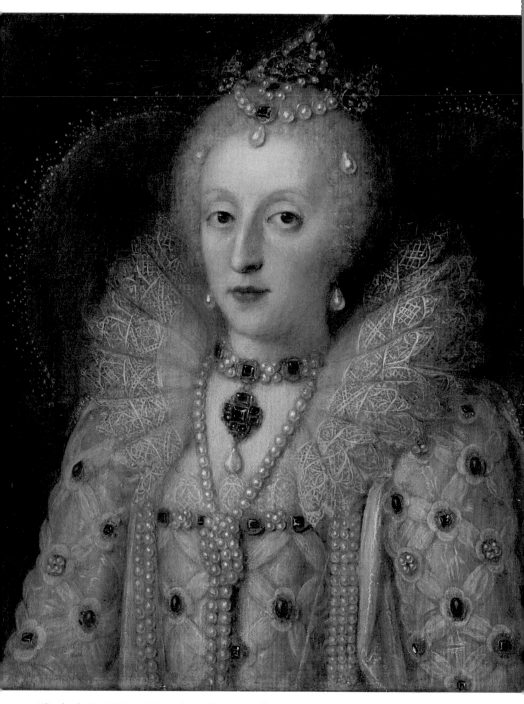

Elizabeth I (1533–1603), whose face was famously damaged by her heavy make-up. (Courtesy of Rijksmuseum)

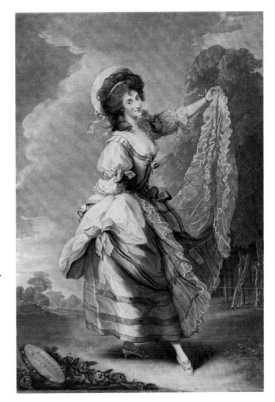

Right: Giovanna Baccelli, dancer, painted by Thomas Gainsborough in ballet pose, 1784. One art critic noted the work was a particularly skilful portrait because the subject was in full stage make-up and 'the face of this admirable artist is evidently *paint-painted*.' (Courtesy of the Yale Center for British Art)

Below: 'Six Stages of Mending a Face, Dedicated with respect to the Right Hon-ble Lady Archer' by Thomas Rowlandson, 29 May 1792. This etching mocks the lengths to which an ageing socialite will go to preserve the appearance of youth; Lady Sarah Archer was well known for her heavy use of cosmetics. (Courtesy of the Metropolitan Museum of Art, Elisha Whittelsey Collection)

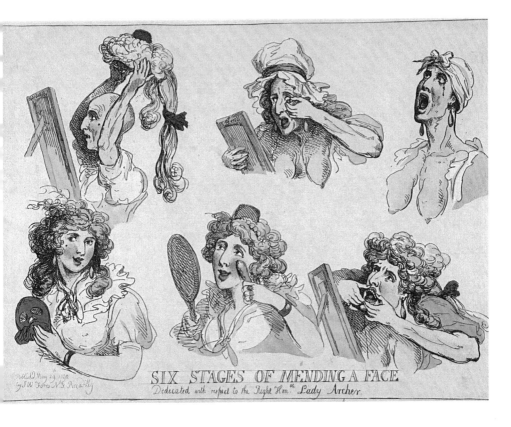

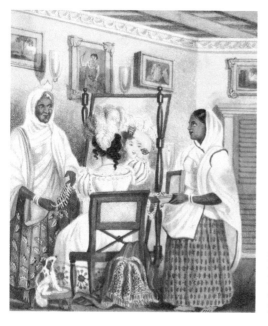

Female Attendants by Sir Charles D'Oyly, nineteenth century, showing an English lady with two Indian attendants. (Courtesy of the Yale Center for British Art)

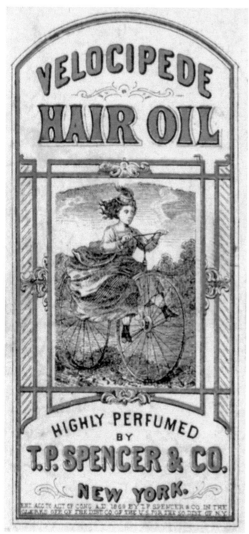

Advertisement for 'Velocipede hair oil, highly perfumed by T.P. Spencer & Co', *c.* 1869. (Courtesy of the Library of Congress)

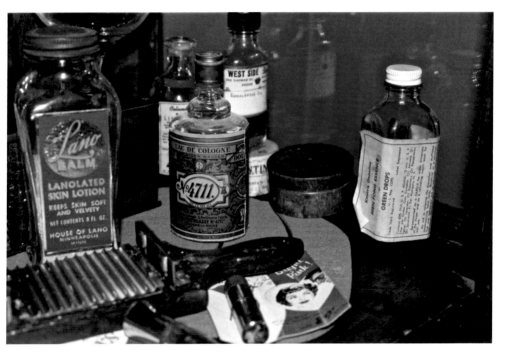

Some original containers from LBCC Historical. Shown here are 4711 Eau De Cologne (1930s); Knorr's Genuine Green Drops (1970s); West Side Pharmacy Eucalyptus Oil, Flame-Glo Triple-Stay Lipstick Bright Pink (1959), Jewel Color Irresistible Lipstick (1966), Dr. Chase's Tooth Dentine Powder Wooden container (early 1900s), Lano Balm Skin Lotion (1940s), wooden piping board used to form pills (1860s). More LBCC Historical items can be found at litttlebits.etsy.com.

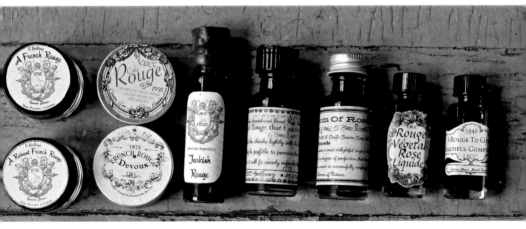

These rouges were all created by LBCC Historical using original recipes from various time periods thoughout history. Left to right, top: 1745 French Rouge; 1931 Cake Rouge; 1810 Turkish Rouge; 1772 A Rouge that Exactly Imitates Nature; 1780-1958 Liquid Bloom of Roses (the longest-running rouge in history); 1922 Rouge Vegetal Rose Liquid; 1849 A Rouge To Give A Beautiful Complexion. The bottom left are 1745 A Robust French Rouge and 1875 French Devoux Rouge. (LBCC)

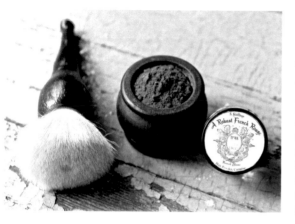

A reproduced cosmetic brush dating from the first half of the eighteenth century and a reproduced wooden rouge pot with an original rouge made from a 1745 recipe by Hannah Glasse. By the late seventeenth century doctors were already aware of the poisons of mercury and lead and were attempting to sway men and women away from those ingredients, primarily by publishing recipes in cookbooks that used all-natural ingredients one would obtain from the local apothecary. (LBCC)

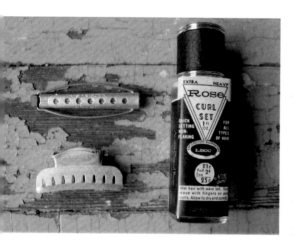

Rose Scented Curling Fluid enhanced the texture, definition and suppleness of setting in curls and waves, and made naturally curly or permed hair easier to manage. It also worked well for fine or thin hair for setting in the marcel waves popular in the 1930s. The Tip-Top Curler (top) was used in the 1930s and 1940s with the curl set. The Tip-Top Marcel Wave Clip (bottom) was used from the 1920s to the 1940s. Tip-Top was a Nebraska company that started out producing parts for the Ford Motor Company before changing to hair-goods production. (LBCC)

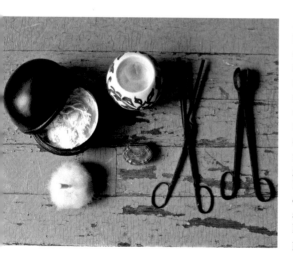

A 1770s powder box (shown open, left) with hair powder made from an original eighteenth-century recipe; a reproduction blue-and-white pomatum (pomade) jar filled with original recipe scented pomatum from 1772 (middle); original eighteenth-century curling tongs (right) and original eighteenth-century papillote curling tongs (far right); original eighteenth-century ivory goose down powderpuff (bottom left). Pomade and hair powder acted as a conditioner and dry shampoo, which allowed women to keep clean hair and have the volume needed to obtain the popular tall hairstyles. (LBCC)

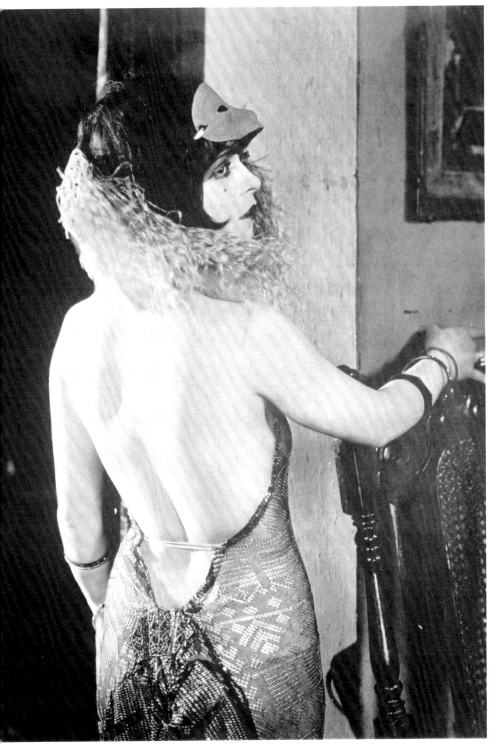

Clara Bow, silent movie actress and vamp, 1920s. That profile could almost be from an Ancient Egyptian tomb. (Courtesy of the Library of Congress)

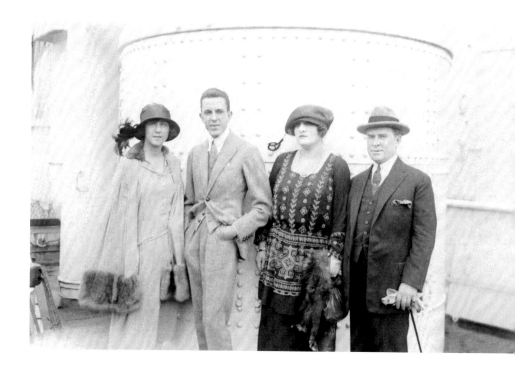

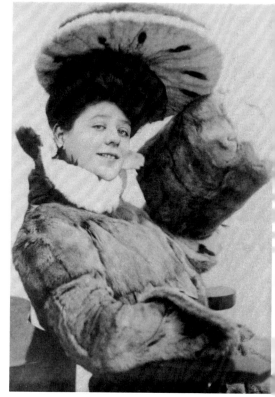

Above: French perfumer Francois Coty (first from left) with his wife (left). In 1904 Coty founded the beauty products manufacturer bearing his name. Today its brands include Calvin Klein, Davidoff and Rimmel. (Courtesy of the Library of Congress)

Right: The Gibson Girl, Camille Clifford, *c.* 1910–15. The Belgian-born Camille won a magazine competition to find the real-life representation of illustrator Charles Gibson's 'ideal woman'; which apparently meant towering hair and an 18-inch waist. (Courtesy of the Library of Congress)

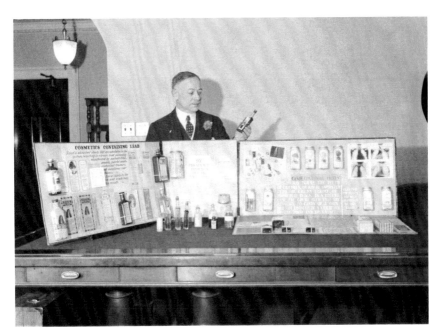

A display of cosmetics containing lead, 1934. (Courtesy of the Library of Congress)

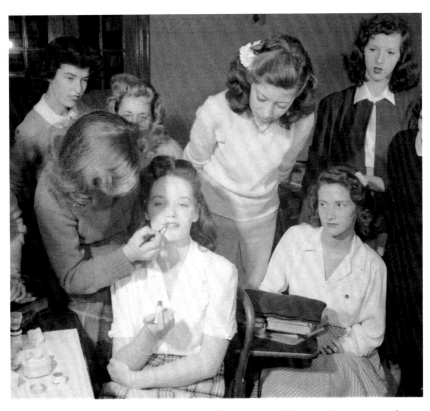

A demonstration of the correct procedure in applying make-up in a home management class at Woodrow Wilson High School, Washington D.C, 1943. (Courtesy of the Library of Congress)

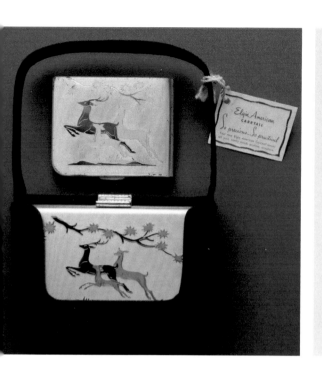

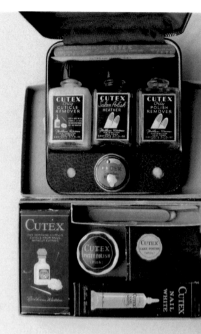

Above left: Elgin American deer compact and bag. (Makeupmuseum.org)

Above right: Cutex manicure set. (Makeupmuseum.org)

Bottom: Avon ice cream lip pomades, 1970s. (Makeupmuseum.org)

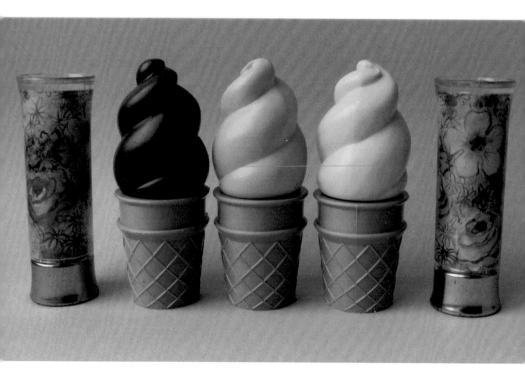

judgements, though the pressure to act irrationally was often put upon them by men, and this spawned literature that included Madame Rachel as a character under thinly-veiled cover – the novel *Lady Audley's Secret* by Wilkie Collins, for example, as well as a number of music hall songs and satirical pieces. It seems that cosmetics, an art form in itself, became a theme in other art forms. Madame Rachel herself, meanwhile, ended her days in a debtors' prison.

Fact in Fiction: Cosmetics and the Nineteenth-Century Novel

The 'penny dreadful', a scandalous magazine that could be purchased cheaply by the ordinary public, serialised stories in which make-up played an important role. Cosmetics often played a part of the plot line of the nineteenth century novel too. The novel as a genre was apt to reflect the Victorian obsession with material culture, dealing with themes such as materiality, artificiality, crime and poison, entrapment into marriage and the supposed gullibility of women. In the story lines, women might be represented as under pressure to preserve their beauty to be socially accepted or ridiculed in their attempts to do so.

In his novel *Armadale*, Wilkie Collins takes cosmetics and the criminality of cosmetics as a theme. The central character, Lydia Gwilt, is an innocent young girl corrupted by an older bawd, much in the style of the female characters that interact in Roman comedy. In this case, Lydia Gwilt is modelled on the infamous Madeline Smith while her older advisor Mother Oldershaw may have been based on Madame Rachel. The story revolves around a husband who, in many ways, is not what his new wife is led to believe. He has indirectly caused the death of his first wife who, through her use of cosmetics in an attempt to beautify herself for him, has died as a result. His second wife goes under cover to find out the truth by wearing make-up. She first finds some cosmetics in her husband's s room that he has used to conceal his own flaws. Beyond hair pomade or a beard or moustache dye, cosmetics were not deemed appropriate for respectable Victorian gentlemen. The husband, on the other hand, may want his wife to look beautiful even when older, while at the same time he fears being deceived,

> You go to the marriage-shop, and get a wife. You take her on the understanding—let us say—that she has lovely yellow hair, that she has an exquisite complexion, that her figure is the perfection of plumpness, and that she is just tall enough to carry the plumpness off. You bring her home, and you discover that it's the old story of the sugar all over again. Your wife is an adulterated article. Her lovely yellow hair is—dye. Her exquisite skin is—pearl powder. Her plumpness is—padding. And three inches of her height are—in the boot-maker's heels. Shut your eyes, and swallow your adulterated wife as you swallow your adulterated sugar— and, I tell you again, you are one of the few men who can try the marriage experiment with a fair chance of success.

Cosmetics are at the centre of the husband and wife relationship in Wilkie Collins' story. In Oscar Wilde's novel *The Picture of Dorian Gray*, cosmetics are again devices to conceal the true character; more than that, the idea of outward beauty concealing immoral character is central to this story. In the character of Dorian Gray, outward beauty conceals pure evil within.

In Louisa May Alcott's novel *Rose in Bloom*, a work somewhat less well-known than her classic *Little Women*, the author demonstrates how experimenting with a new product could turn out to be a risky business in the nineteenth century. In this instance it leads one character in her story, that is Aunt Clara, not being able to attend a ball.

Aunt Clara could not go, for a certain new cosmetic, privately used to improve the once fine complexion which had been her pride till late hours impaired it had brought out an unsightly eruption reducing her to the depths of woe and leaving her no solace for her disappointment but the sight of the elegant velvet dress spread forth upon her bed in melancholy state.

This was a situation that readily occurred in real life.

Manners, etiquette and securing a good marriage are central to the storylines of Jane Austen's novels. The appearance of the women in her various works of fiction does not go unnoticed. Temporary drastic measures might even be taken in order to appear appropriate in front of a guest. The eccentric Mrs Bennet in *Pride and Prejudice* resorts to pinching her cheeks to give them colour in just such a situation. When it comes to falling short of accepted standards in appearance, even the delightful Elizabeth Bennet, whose romantic relationship with the enigmatic Mr Darcy is the book's central theme does not escape some criticism. Caroline Bingley exclaims 'How very ill Eliza Bennet looks this morning Mr Darcy. I never in my life saw any one so much altered as she is since the winter. She is grown so brown and coarse Louisa and I were agreeing that we should not have known her again'. Thankfully Mr Darcy takes a more pragmatic view and puts his down simply to a bit too much sun.

In Austen's novel *Persuasion* Sir Walter, the father of one of the central characters named Anne, attempts to give her some advice as to how to maintain her good looks,

In the course of the same morning, Anne and her father chancing to be alone together, he began to compliment her on her improved looks: he thought her, less thin in her person, in her cheeks; her skin, her complexion, greatly improved: clearer, fresher. Had she been using any thing in particular? — 'No, nothing.' 'Merely Gowland,' he supposed. — 'No, nothing at all.' 'Ha!' he was surprised at that; and added, "Certainly you cannot do better than continue as you are; you cannot be better than well; or I should recommend Gowland, the constant use of Gowland, during the spring months. Mrs. Clay has been using it at my recommendation, and you see what it has done for her. You see how it has carried away her freckles.

This is all very tongue in cheek. Sir Walter is a foolish man and Mrs Clay is another idiotic character in the novel. Austen appears to have understood that Gowland's lotion, a face cream for removing blemishes that was made from lead and mercury, was in fact a dangerous chemical solution that would disfigure rather than improve the complexion. Invented by John Gowland in 1740 for one Elizabeth Chudleigh for blotches, it was basically a corrosive chemical peel. The use of cosmetics is not restricted to women in Austen's novels. In her unfinished novel *The Watsons,* Miss Austen describes Robert Watson a respectable solicitor, making his apologies for his appearance thus; 'We got here so late that I had not time even to put a little fresh powder in my hair'.

Influential Women

The list of nineteenth century women of influence includes Lola Montez (1818–1861), the mistress of the composer Liszt and Louis I of Bavaria, who claimed to be Spanish when in fact she was Irish and, once married, became the Countess of Lansfield. Lola was a powerful trendsetter in respect of women's fashion, especially cosmetics, and wrote a book entitled *The Art and Secrets of Beauty* in 1858, shortly before her death. Cosmetics may have been a factor in her death (by paralysis) although she promoted natural cosmetics in keeping with the notions of the time. As I have mentioned, Queen Alexandra (1844–1925), the glamorous wife of Edward VII, was known for enamelling her face. Edward, after all, was attracted to the painted ladies of the theatre. Perhaps in an effort to compete for his attentions, Alexandra wore cosmetics at evening functions and as a result was accused of flaunting herself through her use of obvious make-up, which she set off with violet perfume, her signature scent. The wives of diplomats, even women adventurers, brought back ideas to Europe from further afield. Those who wrote about their travels, for example, Mary Elizabeth Rodgers, the sister of a British Official who spent two years in Palestine, admired the pale beauty of women in Eastern harems.

The Seven Sutherland Sisters

The seven Sutherland sisters were born into abject poverty in New York between 1851 and 1865. Their father, a church minister, had them perform as a cabaret act to make money. Their singing performance was rather unremarkable, and of much less interest than the length of their hair. At the end of their act, their father would call, 'Let down your hair'. Victorian ladies wore their hair up and long hair was considered very erotic. Each of the Sutherland sisters had hair that measured at least 5 feet or more. The Victorians had a strange liking for people exhibiting themselves and the seven Sutherland sisters' father saw a business opportunity not only in the show per se but also in marketing a hair tonic. The girls appeared to be living proof that the mixture of witch hazel, water, rum, salt, magnesium and hydrochloric acid, worked. One of the sisters, Naomi, married the son of Bailey, of Barnum and Bailey's circus. The said Henry Bailey was able to help market the Sutherland Sisters and their products in order to make this a vibrant business. After the death of their father, the girls became owners of the company and branched out into other cosmetics including hair colorants, scalp cleansers and face creams. In an age when men and women often lost their hair not only through aging but on account of illness and their use of harsh abrasive products, the Sutherland girls' long hair was much to be envied. It seemed that long hair might even be an indication of the presence of magical powers particularly as there were seven sisters and the number seven has always been linked with the supernatural. The nineteenth century was an age especially susceptible to such ideas.

Popular Products

Beasley's druggist (1853) recommends Orfila's Hair Dye, a potentially lethal concoction,

> Take three parts of litharge and two of quicklime, both impalpable powder, and mix them carefully. When used, a portion of the powder is mixed with hot water or milk, and applied to the hair, the part being afterwards enveloped in oil-skin, or a cabbage-leaf, for four or five hours.

The use of this product was likely to result in hair loss and over the longer-term damage to the internal organs. At least some hair dye products carried warnings of the dangers of frequent use. Condy's Fluid was one such pigment. Applied to darken the hair and cover grey, advertisements claimed that 'Condy's Fluid is sometimes efficacious; but it is not well to use it too often'. Made from a mixture of potassium permanganate and common table salt, sodium chloride, this was put to use not only as a hair dye but as a disinfectant and as a deodorant. As a hair dye it was recommended that this be applied carefully and used to cover only small amounts of grey so as not permanently stain and harm the skin. Applying it to the hair was sometimes done with a toothbrush, strand by strand, so it was not only a dangerous but a laborious procedure. Even the salt might cause skin irritation upon drying. An application of Condy's fluid consisted of two teaspoonfuls of the fluid itself mixed with cold breakfast tea and an herbal tea made from rosemary. After washing or shampooing, the roots of the hair were retouched with this liquid using a small sponge.

According to *The London News* (1892), 'The beauty of the skin is enhanced by *Poudre d'amour*'. Available in three colours, *Blanche, Naturelle* and Rachel, at the cost of 1s, this product claimed to soften and beautify the skin of ladies, and soothe the male skin after shaving. The tints catered for fair and darker skin while the shade called Rachel was deemed suitable for wearing in artificial light. The colour Rachel was probably named after a famous French actress Eliza Rachel Felix, whose beauty was renowned, rather than after the infamous con artist Madame Rachel. The product could be bought at various outlets but also purchased by post. *Poudre D'Amour* came in the form of sheets, contained in a small book. These could be used discreetly to take the shine off one's nose or conceal a blemish. Powdered papers like this are still on sale today. The name *Poudre D'Amour* not only evoked an image of fashionable Paris but implied by using this that love would follow and that the lady would get her man. Advertisements for the product visually reinforced this suggestion.

Pearl powder was all the rage if you could afford it. Saltwater pearls were expensive, but pearls from fresh oysters, or mother of pearl from the shells, could be ground down to make a face powder. Colin Mackenzie in his book *Five Thousand Receipts in all the Useful and Domestic Arts* (1829) recommended that a good chemist should stock the real thing 'for the curious and the rich'. If pearls were too expensive or scarce, then an alternative was bismuth, a naturally occurring grey white metallic powder. John Churchill, chemist, notes two alternative recipes dating from 1841: 'Take pearl of bismuth white and French chalk equal parts. Reduce them to a fine powder and sift through lawn', or

'Take one pound of bismuth one ounce of starch powder and one ounce of orris powder. Mix and sift them through lawn. Add a drop of attar of roses or neroli'. The second recipe with its large portion of bismuth may be somewhat more toxic, while the first recipe is somewhat more diluted. The latter has the added attraction of a pleasant smell.

Eau de Lis was, according to *Beauty Culture* (1898),

> ...made from the genuine recipe used by the lovely *Ninon de L'Enclos*, the beautiful Lola Montez, and the beauties of the court of Charles II of England, is a soothing wash which prevents wrinkles and crow's-feet, obviates undue flushing, keeps the skin fresh and smooth, and is invaluable in hot climates.

This advertisement for *Eau de Lis* promises much but gives little away as to its contents. This is also a good example of how a lineage, and therefore credibility, could be established for a product by a spot of name dropping to indicate use by renowned society beauties in order to establish its place as a product tried and tested over time, making it 'a must have' for any lady of fashion.

Hazeline Snow was a so-called vanishing cream that first appeared on the market in 1892. An oil-in-water mixture made from stearic acid, (a natural component of butter, tallow and animal fats in general) combined with a polyol, an alcohol compound, and water, the product got its name from the fact that it appeared to vanish when applied to the skin. Not only was Hazeline Snow easily absorbed but it also felt pleasant, soothing and softening the skin. It left an attractive pearly sheen too, which suggested glamour. Up until the end of World War I when so called 'vanishing creams' fell out of fashion, many cosmetics companies manufactured products such as this.

Rice powder had long been used to whiten the face as well as for powdering wigs. By the end of the nineteenth century, named products based on rice powder such as *Poudre de Riz de Java* began to appear. There were many powders allegedly made from rice powder but even if labelled as such, these were often made from more dangerous substances. In a report on face powders (1897) doctor, pharmacologist and toxicologist William Murrell found that 'face powders commonly employed for the complexion no longer consisted of powdered rice but were combinations in various proportions of chalk, white lead, bismuth common starch and alabaster'.

An advertisement in the journal *Home Notes* (1895) shows a group of woman sharing a secret. That secret was the means of achieving

> ...the most lovely complexion that the imagination could desire; clear, fresh, free from blotch, blemish, coarseness, redness, freckles or pimples. One box of Dr MacKenzies improved harmless arsenic wafers Post free for 4s.6d. Beware of injurious imitations.

Although referred to as a wafer, this was in fact an easily dissolving pill. In America, the same product was advertised under the names of Rose, Simms and Campbell, all apparently medical men. These tablets, composed of arsenic, were ingested to produce a clear complexion. They were bought in boxes, sometimes alongside a soap also made of arsenic that would appear to work with the tablets. The effect of taking such a product would be to kill off one's red blood cells, which would certainly have made a lady look pale. The word 'safe' regularly features in the adverts for this product. Though the dangers of arsenic were known there was a school of thought there was some benefit in consuming it.

Bloom of Ninon was the name of a product popular in the eighteenth century and comprised of some very dangerous ingredients; the nineteenth century *Bloom of Ninon* inherited the name but not the ingredients. This was a Victorian face powder made from chalk, talcum powder, bismuth, zinc oxide and starch and scented of orris and rose.

Advertisements for Empress Josephine's face bleach promised a much sought after pale and blemish free complexion and contained many an endorsement by well known society ladies, as well as bearing the name of the Empress Josephine herself. The very name suggested that perfect beauty was within a woman's grasp should she just apply this mixture. A further more sinister clue to its composition is also in the name. This was indeed bleach, a mixture of lead carbonate, mercury and zinc, and using it risked a range of serious physical and neurological symptoms – and even death. Although companies advertising these products were at pains to stress that these were safe to use, given the knowledge of the dangers of the ingredients of many of these products, it is surprising that they were so popular.

Alternatively... Some Recipes to Make at Home
A skin lightening recipe or 'Pearl water for the face':

> Put half a pound of the best Spanish oil soap which has been cut or scraped very fine into a gallon of boiling water. Stir the whole well for some time then let it stand till cold. Now add quart of rectified spirits of wine and half an ounce of oil of rosemary stirring the whole well together.
>
>

The British Perfumer

Wrinkle lotions to be painted on thrice daily:

1 ½ tannin, 7 oz rosewater 3 oz glycerine, ½ ounce eau-de-cologne, Or 1 oz lemon juice, 1 oz eau- de- cologne 1 oz simple tincture of benzoin and 2oz distilled water.

Beauty Culture

Hair Dye

Most of the dyes sold for the hair are caustic and should be used with great care. it not infrequently happened by mismanagement that one head of hair appears half a dozen shades of colour. the following receipts are quite new and from good authority: any of the articles may be bought at the druggists. Take one pint common wine, two drams common salt, four drams green copper; boil for some minutes and then add oxide of copper two drams: boil for two minutes take from the fire and add four drams powdered nut galls. Rub the hair with this composition and some moments afterwards.

Ladies Guide to Perfect Gentility

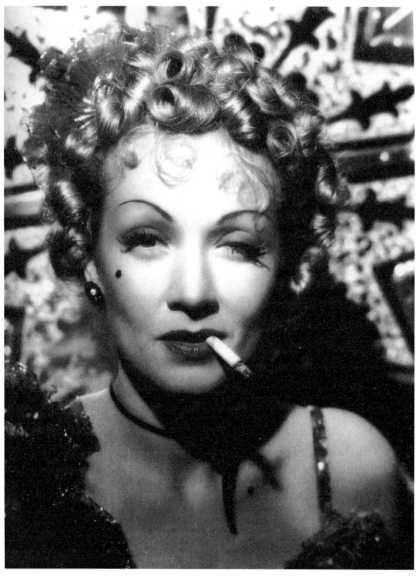

Marlene Dietrich. (Author's collection)

'I dress for the image. Not for myself, not for the public,
not for fashion, not for men.'

8

THE TWENTIETH CENTURY:

THE MAGIC OF THE MOVIES, MAKE-UP AND THE WAR EFFORT, AND MASS MEDIA ADVERTISING

The greatest fun of all is the making up, which takes at least six hours. Strong astringent first to tighten one's face... liquid powder, rouge. Best black for the eyelashes, turquoise grease for the lids, vermillion for the eyes and for the nostrils, carmine for the lips...

Cecil Beaton, fashion photographer

Introduction

Two World Wars, female emancipation, the influence of cinema, the advent of television and the invention of the motor car all had implications for make-up, not only in terms of what was available but also with regard to how it was worn. At the beginning of the century the use of cosmetics was largely discreet. Heavy make-up continued to be associated with the theatre, with actresses and other women of low status or ill repute, though the suffragettes challenged this notion by defiantly wearing bright red lipstick in their campaign for female emancipation. Paris had long had a number of specialist beauty shops openly offering treatments and products (as opposed to the back door establishments of Madame Rachel or Frances Henning) and these began to appear in London and in New York in the first decade of the twentieth century.

However some powders and rouges might still be made at home. *The Dudley Recipe Book of Cookery and Household Recipes,* collected and arranged by Georgiana Countess of Dudley and published in 1910, contains a few cosmetic recipes (a rosemary hair wash and a recipe for cold cream for example), but, aside from the shortages that occurred during World War II in particular, cosmetics were increasingly commercially manufactured and shop bought. World War II brought a boom in advertising and, once rationing was over, a large variety of beauty products for which there was considerable demand, flooded the market. While many remained expensive, there were other cheaper options so no one went without. By the middle of the twentieth century, cosmetics had become big business. Celebrities of stage and screen and other prominent female figures in public life became role models, seen everywhere not only on film and in the theatre but also on billboards and in magazines. Their appearance was copied by the woman in the street. Cosmetic firms began to make large profits. In the latter half of the twentieth century, new technologies in the production of cosmetics as well as mass media advertising encouraged continually changing and evolving fashions in terms of the look women were trying to achieve, whether that was the wide-eyed innocence of model Twiggy or pouting lips of actress Sophia Loren. One of the most fundamental changes was the popularity of a tan.

Men got in on the act too. Popular male musicians in the 1970s began to use make-up to create an alter ego or persona as part of their on stage acts – think of David Bowie and his spaceman, or the distinctive eye make-up of Alice Cooper. Make-up became associated with particular genres of music, in particular heavy metal and punk rock. The cosmetic formed a part of visual entertainment of their stage shows, self-identity and a further dimension to the kind of music being performed. By the end of the century, make-up for male musicians was discreet, if used at all, but in real life more skin care products specifically for men had appeared on the market.

After the wide range of colours of colours worn in the 1950s, and more specifically the psychedelic colours in the '60s, the fashion for the natural look again became the ideal for women. Manufacturers had to take an ethical approach to the production of make-up in response to public concern about animal testing and environmental issues; naturally sourced cosmetics *per se*, and not just a natural look, were in. By the end of the twentieth century, whether particular cosmetics were intended for women or for men, the manufacturers increasingly claimed that these could effect something more than skin deep and could benefit one's overall health, harking back to days of Ancient Egypt, Greece and Rome when health and make-up had been, to all intents and purposes, indistinguishable.

The Edwardians

At the beginning of the twentieth century, city dwellers lived in a generally unhealthy environment. Smog was a particular problem for those living in the larger industrialised conurbations and this was telling on the skin. Air pollution caused people to age faster. However, this was not the only danger to the well-being of the population. The Edwardians' high carbohydrate diet and their general lack of exercise played havoc with their health and, as a result, their appearance. An outbreak of tuberculosis at the beginning of the century perpetuated the fashion for the pale and frail look that had been appreciated by the Victorians. For a short time, it was still chic to look sick. In some quarters cosmetics were still strongly disapproved of, and their use cited as an example of the foolishness of female character. Women did try to keep their complexions young and fresh by applying creams and drinking lemon juice to affect that pale complexion. A hint of a blush was always considered attractive so light rouge was popular and widely available. Powdered sheets of papers were pressed against the cheek to give a hint of colour and rice powder was applied to give a pearly glow.

Cosmetic surgery was something new, in the modern world at least; the ancient Egyptians had been quite adept at attaching prosthetic toes or correcting a crooked nose. One newspaper carried the following report: 'The Derma Featural Company sued in the Westminster County Court a youth named Spence for £15 15s ... being the balance due for "building up a new nose".' The defendant, who pleaded infancy, was ordered to pay 5s weekly. Clearly the abilities of whoever carried out this particular operation were not up to scratch. This is hardly surprising as the cosmetic surgery was unregulated and it seems from this case that there was no age restriction on who could give consent.

The Power of Lipstick

Over the centuries women had felt the pressure to attain a high standard of attractiveness and although they might compete with each other to achieve that standard, it was in essence set by the opposite sex. Cosmetics might still be worn as an aid to achieving perfection, provided her powder and paint was applied well and out of sight of men. However, those fighting to improve the social and political lot of women at the beginning of the twentieth century had begun to change things. Not only did the suffragettes sport daring bright red lipstick but the lipstick case took on the shape of bullets, reminiscent of the bullet casings used in the World War One. This was women at war fighting for their political and civil rights, using make-up as a weapon. Cosmetics made a statement about the rejection of male domination and signalled personal freedom.

It was in 1915 that an American, Maurice Levy, invented the container for lipstick that we recognise today. Lipstick began to be mass-produced and its popularity quickly grew. The basic ingredients of a lipstick at this time consisted of wax, a pigment and an emollient. Poucher in his *Perfumes Cosmetics and Soaps*, a standard reference book on make-up for the industry in print since 1923, stated, in the 1926 edition, that 'lipsticks have gained popularity during the past ten years to such an extent that they are now probably used more than any other single cosmetic product'. Lip gloss dyed with bromo acid to create a pink-red shade was made popular by the actress Lillian Gish. The range of colours available grew and grew. The True Red favoured by the suffragettes was joined by other shades of red to suit different hair colours. Pastel shades in rose pink and coral were also introduced. The Tangee lipstick was first manufactured in 1922 by a company of that name in Vermont in the United States. This was a very popular brand reinventing itself to take account of changing trends in fashion and lifestyle. However, in 1924, the reader might be surprised to learn that The New York Board of Health thought about banning lipstick, fearing that it could possible poison the men who kissed the women who wore it. Fear of women gaining power and influence over men, a fear which was, in part at least, responsible for the high standards of beauty, appears in this instance seems to have raised its head again. However, this isn't perhaps quite as silly as it sounds. Dangerous substances such as lead, mercury, arsenic and vermillion had been used in lipstick and although these poisons were meant, by this time, to be a thing of the past, even in the twenty first century questions are still asked about the composition of lipstick, such as the possible presence of lead, for example. In the 1930s one daily paper remarked that lipsticks were going out of fashion due to the high cost of removing lipstick stains from clothing. However, in 1953 advertisements for the still popular Tangee brand claimed that their lipstick, which was lanolin based and made from only natural ingredients, stayed in place not only when you eat or kiss but also if you smoke. Lipstick on a collar need no longer disclose an illicit affair nor could a lipstick-stained cigarette spoil the sense of style and glamour associated with smoking promoted by Hollywood movie stars, who were regularly seen with a cigarette both on and off the screen. From 1931, lipsticks had been widely on sale in shops from the ubiquitous Woolworths at the cheaper end of the market to the more exclusive department stores. Lipsticks were given increasingly adventurous names, generally recalling food or drink or with allusion to sex or romance: Black Honey, Truly Toffee, Lady Danger, Girl About Town and Strawberry Fizz, to name but a few.

The Roaring Twenties

An article titled 'Flapper Jane', which appeared in the magazine *The New Republic* in 1925 describes the twenties flapper in somewhat unflattering terms. Flapper girls were heavily made up

> not to imitate nature but for an altogether artificial effect – pallor mortis, poisonously scarlet lips, richly ringed eyes –the later looking not so much debauched (which is the intention) as diabetic.

Silent movie actresses including Theda Bara, Mary Pickford, Clara Bow and Louise Brooks sported large dark eyes, prominent lips and slicked back hair These icons of style, known as vamps, short for vampires, played exotic, sometimes semi-erotic roles in the films in which they appeared. Theda Bara, for example, played the parts of Queen Cleopatra and the temptress Salome. Young women adopted this style of make-up with the androgynous clothing that reflected their new-found freedoms. Although vamp make-up on screen looked very dark if one compares the film material with the coloured images of movie stars on magazine covers, it seems that while the make up was heavy it was often golden brown in tone. The cinema techniques used at the time distorted the depth of the shades. The alteration made to colour by early techniques in cinematography would again present problems when films began to be shot in colour.

In the 1920s and '30s, beauties advertised cosmetics, lending the products they endorsed an air of sophistication and class. Lady Diana Manners (the daughter of the 8th Duke of Rutland and his wife Violet) was a well-known socialite and the wife to the British ambassador to France. Diana's great beauty is described in detail in advertisements where she endorses Ponds Cold Cream; 'and the lily's own petals are not more snowy white more satin soft than Lady Diana's skin'. The language and the comparisons made are very similar to those used by the Roman authors such as Ovid and Propertius so many centuries before. Sometimes it seems with regard to make-up remarkably little had changed.

Art and Artistry; Art Deco and the Ballets Russes

Bringing to mind Japanese prints, the Art Deco movement, dominated Western Europe and America, influencing styles not only in painting, pottery and other artistic media but also in make-up with its sharp, well-defined lines and use of blocks of bright colour. Styles in hats for women, which shielded the face, also drew attention to the eyes, which were heavily painted with pencil lines and the newly invented mascara. Vaseline on the eyelids attracted light. The visits to Europe of Diaghilev's Ballets Russes also nurtured enthusiasm for dramatic eye make-up and all things oriental. The dancers wore exaggerated make-up with much Eastern kohl around their eyes in keeping with the often oriental looking costumes designed for them by the king of fashion or *la magnifique* as he was known in Paris, the one and only Paul Poiret. Poiret, who had business interests across the world of fashion, had his own perfume and cosmetics company too (established in 1911) which he called Rosine after his eldest daughter.

All Things Egyptian

On 4 November 1922 Howard Carter made his now famous discovery, the tomb of the Ancient Egyptian boy king Tutankhamen. Interest in the ancient past was not new. After all, the silent movie actress Theda Bara had appeared in seductive pose in the 1917 movie about Cleopatra, silent movies had been brought to the screen featuring Helen of Troy, Julius Caesar, and the excitement of chariot racing in *Ben Hur*, and contemporary ideas of beauty still harked back to the classical world. The discovery of Tutankhamen's tomb, however, fired even greater interest in the history of Ancient Egypt in particular. In a more concrete connection between past and present, toilette artefacts had been found in the boy king's tomb. Indeed, the seductive scent of some of these ancient perfumes and ointments had even been fleetingly sensed by Carter and his fellow archaeologists when they opened Tutankhamen's burial place. Elaborate containers, some made of alabaster, gold, or encrusted with precious stones, were an indication of their treasured contents. One such jar was found to contain a perfumed ointment made from animal fat resin and spikenard, an expensive plant that grew not in Egypt but in the higher reaches of the Himalayas. This was indeed a scented ointment fit for a king. The famous gold mask of Tutankhamen as well as other images of him clearly shows the line of kohl eye make-up that both Egyptian men and women wore as protection from the sun and sand. All things Egyptian were suddenly very much in fashion, and the ancient Egyptian trend for wearing make-up, particularly eye make-up which, although it had now lost its association with religion and superstition, crops up again as a point of fashion. The fascination with Ancient Egypt continued, fuelled by the remaking of the movie *Antony and Cleopatra* in

1963, staring Elizabeth Taylor and Richard Burton. The lavish set, Miss Taylor's own iconic beauty as well as her torrid love affair, on and off screen with Burton, served to draw attention to the striking make-up. However it would not be until the end of the century that researchers established that eye make-up had probably been worn by the Ancient Egyptian to protect their eyes from heat and dust, and therefore infection, and not only for aesthetic reasons.

Cosmetic Containers, Practical and Luxurious

In the twentieth century, make-up made a serious move out of the privacy of the bedroom into public areas such as hotel lounges, theatre foyers and other public venues. Society ladies in the 1930s often carried a *minaudiere*, a small metal plated accessory attractively decorated with, for example, semi precious stones. This object hung on a short chain and was just big enough to store a lipstick, rouge, make up and powder. The new portability of make-up allowed those who were not averse to doing so, to touch up their make-up in public –even though many people disapproved of this. In 1924, an American advertisement for Pond's Cold Cream explained the important of cosmetic creams (and indeed cosmetics in general) to the increasingly large numbers of young female office workers with the tag line 'girls in business are as fresh and lovely at five as at nine'. The advertisement blames 'clattering typewriters', dust and 'responsibilities that bring tired lines of worry' for destroying a girl's looks. However, according to Pond's promotional material, at least this was something that could be rectified if the unfortunate office worker only had their product to hand. There was a wide range of make-up on the market adaptable for wear from daytime into evening and to suit every hair colour and complexion. Blurring the idea of gendered space, in the early days this could literally stop the traffic as men in particular turned to look at something that had previously been hidden behind closed doors. At home on her dressing table, a wealthy socialite might display expensive boxes, bottles and jars. Exclusive French designers, such as Lalique and Baccarat, specialists in glassware, and saw an opportunity. The stylish bottles they made for the perfume and cosmetics industry are still, in their own right, much sought after today.

Cosmetics: *The Secret of a Happy Marriage*

In the first half of the twentieth century at least, it was as important as ever for women to make efforts to appeal to and conform to what their male counterparts found attractive. This could cement their future in terms of marriage and financial security. Spinsterhood did not appeal to the majority of women. From the early years of the twentieth century up until the 1960s we find newspaper and magazine articles claiming that a woman's appearance secures her a long and happy marriage while neglect of her person does not. In 1929, the Reuter's News Agency quoted Miss Frances Martell of Chicago who claimed, in a address to a convention of the National Association of Cosmeticians, that 'the woman who gets the most attention from her husband is the one whose cheeks are pink, whose lips are vermillion and whose nails are newly manicured'. According to Miss Martell, 'nine tenths of husbands cited in divorce cases are married to drab wives'. *The London Opinion Magazine* carries the same sorry message in its October edition in 1954. 'In nine out of ten cases when a marriage broke down it was fundamentally the woman's fault and primarily through failing as a wife to maintain the high standard of personal appearance which she had of herself as a spinster'. This of course pre-dates the birth of the women's liberation movement and the rise of feminism. While it is hard for most of us now to comprehend such a view, think back to the Roman world and the satirist Juvenal to claims that men would discard their wives when they showed signed of aging and the many marriages of convenience made in which, other than being a member of the elite, appearance was the only thing that mattered. It would be end of the twentieth century before the open expression of the idea that beauty was key to a woman's success in life, whether marriage or a good career, became tempered by the worth of women in terms of intellect and ability. Sadly, it would be naive to suggest that looks no longer matter.

Cosmetics for Motoring

Early motor vehicles offered little protection from the elements. *The Scotsman* newspaper carried an article in 1937 entitled 'Look your best while driving: Tips for women motorists'. The article notes: 'How annoying for a woman, after stepping into her car beautifully dressed and carefully made up to discover at the end of the journey that tired lines have appeared round her eyes and her face looks far from clean!' According to this newspaper article, the solution to the damage done by the wind and dust was the application of pure milk, rubbed on with a piece of cotton wool before travelling by car. At the end of the journey, cleansing cream to remove any dirt should discreetly be used. An eye bath of boracic solution was all that was required to prepare a lady's eyes for the journey and wearing dark glasses to prevent squinting in the sunlight was essential. This advice ensured that the lady arrived, as the newspaper assures its readers, as 'fresh as the proverbial daisy'.

The Society Hostess

Advertisers in the early years of the twentieth century found it difficult to persuade women in upper class society to endorse their products but by the '30s this was beginning to change. It was not so much the money but the publicity that these women enjoyed. For example our glamorous society hostess, Lady Diana Cooper (nee Manners), now the wife of the British ambassador to France, promoted Ponds Cold Cream. Gladys, Duchess of Marlborough, also endorsed cold cream. Her beauty had been admired in her youth by Rodin and Proust. She claimed that Ponds Cream helped 'keep her complexion so vigorous and health, and that she never worried about 'windburn and chapping'. Endorsements like these went a long way to increasing sales and earned those who endorsed them an income in the lean years of war time especially. Those in the public eye, like Lady Diana Cooper (nee Manners), also commented on the appearance of other women of note. In one of her letters dated May 1951, Lady Diana gives a description of Wallis Simpson, the controversial future wife of Edward, Prince of Wales, for whom he gave up his right to the throne,

> Wallis had had her hair blue powdered and spangled ... She wore a short expensive white satin dress, looked remarkably fresh and alarmingly overexcited, jitterbugging, talking too fast and too repetitively.

Lights! Camera! Action! Max Factor and Hollywood Glamour

Max Factor was born in Russia and trained as a chemist before beginning his career as a make-up artist in theatre working with the Russian ballet. He emigrated to America in 1904 and within a few years of living in the States, he had opened his own make-up and wig business in Los Angeles. Max began supplying make-up and wigs to the flourishing film business in Hollywood. The cowboys scalped by the Indians in the popular westerns of the day wore wigs hired from Max Factor's shop. The merchandise was so valuable that he often sent his sons along to the film studio to keep an eye on his wigs and to make sure none of them were damaged on set.

On screen at the start of the twentieth century, the faces of the actors and actresses appeared green because early movies were filmed using Technicolor, a means of photographing moving pictures using artificial colour. Max Factor invented a thin greasepaint make-up that corrected this. Through his skilful use of cosmetics, in shades tailored to the individual, Max Factor helped create the look that we associate with many well known actresses; for example, those heart-shaped lips of Clara Bow and Jean Harlow's signature platinum hair colour. Off screen many of the famous actresses of the early movies, including Jean Harlow, Bette Davis and Marlene Dietrich, were customers at his salon. These glamorous women helped to promote his products and make Max Factor world famous as 'make-up artist to the stars'.

When he died in 1938, his sons took over the business, which continued to expand significantly beyond the world of stage and screen. Building on the make-up produced for the movies, pancake make-up was a runaway commercial success. This cosmetic became known as pancake make-up because it was moist or moistened before being applied but did not cake or crack. In later years the company is credited both with manufacturing the first concealer and also with pioneering waterproof make-up. The company, now part of the Proctor & Gamble group, continues to be a well-known player in today's cosmetics industry. The Hollywood Powder Puff War was the name given to the battle between rivals Max Factor and Elizabeth Arden to dominate cosmetics for film. Far from being a trivial dispute, this revolved around important questions not only of money and domination of the industry but also matters of female identity, working practices and matters of race.

Blonde Bombshells

The reclusive American billionaire and inventor Howard Hughes dubbed the glamorous Miss Jean Harlow the platinum blonde. Harlow was well aware of the importance of her hair to her success in film and felt forced to live up to Hughes' description. Painful visits to her hairdresser maintained her hair's signature colour: a sort of white blonde. Although the actress protested that this was her natural colour, her hairdresser Alfred Pagano acknowledged later that the colour was the result of an application of peroxide, ammonia Clorox (an American household cleaner) and Lux flakes; all in all, a truly caustic combination. Her own hair eventually fell out and she was forced to wear a wig. The concoction she had applied to her hair (known as double blonding) probably contributed to her painful death from kidney failure, aged just twenty-six.

Many of Hollywood's biggest stars wore wigs, sometimes as a permanent component of their appearance, and others for particular roles they played. Frank Sinatra wore a toupee, while Marlene Dietrich owned and sported a wig, which she had dusted with twenty carat gold for a sparkling effect. Marilyn Munroe's funerary make-up took three hours and was done as instructed in her will by the cosmetics artist who had made her up in life. Movie stars replaced society ladies advertising and endorsing beauty products. Greta Garbo, for example, popularised eye brow pencils. The Bond movie *Goldfinger* even reintroduced make-up as a murder weapon in quirky fashion when the glamour interest played by Shirley Eaton dies from being completely covered in gold body paint.

The Mysterious Disappearance of Aviation Pioneer Miss Amelia Earhart

The famous aviator Amelia Earhart (1897–1937) disappeared without trace while flying over the Pacific Ocean at the beginning of July 1937 in an attempt to circumnavigate the globe at the equator. Little was known about her disappearance until very recently. New evidence as to her demise came in the form of a jar of Dr Berry's Freckle Ointment, found in fragments on the uninhabited island Nikumaroro ion the South Pacific. It had long been known that this was the area in which Earhart had disappeared. Dr Berry's cream was produced in the early twentieth century and advertised as a mixture that would cause freckles to fade. It was common knowledge that Miss Earhart had freckles and intensely disliked them. The fragments of a product with which she had affinity may be only circumstantial evidence, but is nevertheless intriguing.

World War II; Make-up and the War effort

World War II brought a shortage of make-up that had, between the wars, become all the rage. Supplies became scarce and while some cosmetics were available, they were rationed, taxed and very expensive. Some of the ingredients, tin for example, were needed for the war effort. Cosmetic supplies were used up in wartime factories, making products that could be useful at the front. Coty, for instance, instead of making face powders, switched to foot powders and anti-gas ointment. Cyclax provided a sunscreen, which was used for camouflage, while Elizabeth Arden invented a scar cream, effective in the treatment of burns. Using metal to manufacture powder compacts or lipstick cases was banned in Britain in 1942; what make-up could be had, was available in plain cardboard packaging, sometimes without all its constituent parts such as powder without the powder puff, and lipstick without the casing, in effect, a refill.

Hitler hated make-up. Anti-cosmetic rhetoric abounded in Germany but women still used cosmetics. The composer Wagner's daughter arrived at where his works were being performed, sporting scarlet toenails. German magazines, on the other hand, compromised, advocating discreet use of make-up. The German labour front offered courses in how to apply make-up. Girls had lessons on health and beauty in school, though publicly hair dyes and make-up were discouraged. Spies, that is those working under cover in a country other than their own, were kitted out with make-up appropriate to the country they were working in, in order to complete their disguise.

Make Do and Mend

The culture of 'make do and mend' extended to beauty products, as it did to most things during the war. There was also a thriving black market in whatever fancy goods could be obtained. When things were scarce, rationed or expensive, women used whatever alternatives they could find. They improvised with beetroot juice instead of rouge, and used burnt matchsticks to darken eyelashes. Calamine lotion was mixed with cold cream to create foundation. Cosmetics could still be grown in the garden. Anything made from roses (such as face creams and refreshing floral waters) was believed to be effective and therefore valued. Hair lotions using herbs such as rosemary were also popular. The natural red dye from geraniums or poppy petals stained lips in place of a lipstick. Shortages were a reality but so was increased demand fuelled by the media and even by the government, whose posters of land girls or Wrens showed smiling girls wearing bright lipstick and mascara.

Put on a Brave Face

> Efficiency today is also charming and the Girl at the Wheel can, in a few moments transport her trim self into the loveliest glamour of evening make-up ... with the aid of Cashmere Bouquet.
>
> A newspaper advertisement from 1941

Cosmetics themselves were recognised as an important tool in boosting morale during the war. A woman was encouraged to make the best of herself as part of her personal contribution to the war effort. Colgate's Cashmere Bouquet produced a range of cleansers, foundations, powders, lipstick and rouge aimed at helping women in the war effort by literally 'putting on a brave face' and turning the hardworking girl by day into the perfect partner for a glamorous evening out. Women were expected to move effortlessly from uniform to evening wear, with make-up matching their outfit and the occasion –and in so doing, raise the morale of their men folk. This wasn't easily achieved, but even the government saw a well-groomed woman as a 'morale booster' for both sexes at this difficult time.

Canned Hosiery

Items of clothing such as stockings were scarce and expensive, even if they could be found on the black market. In Britain, women 'made do' using burnt matchsticks to paint lines on their legs to give the illusion of seamed stockings or even staining their legs with Bovril. Women in America turned to products called for example 'stockingless cream' or 'liquid stockings', manufactured by a number of make-up companies including Elizabeth Arden. In fact, this canned hosiery, as it was known, had been available in fashionable London, if not elsewhere in Britain, in 1929. According to the trade journal *The American Perfumer and Essential Oil Review* (1929):

A leading store in the British metropolis is now selling in its toilet goods section a thick, smooth cream which, when spread evenly and generously all over the leg, from ankle to well above the knee, has all the appearance of beautiful silk stockings. It does not crack, it does not irritate the skin (in fact, it prevents sunburn), and it does not rub off until removed with the aid of warm water and soap. This new 'hosiery cream' is sold in large collapsible tubes and in bottles. It is available in many of the latest and most popular silk stocking shades. Women can choose a shade between the palest beige and dark ochre shades. Actresses are using these bottled stockings considerably, so are girls on seaside vacations, and it requires the very closest and repeated inspection to reveal the fact that the limbs are not clothed in the orthodox manner.

Having proved less popular in Britain to begin with, the fashion for cosmetic stockings really caught on as war shortages began to bite. Canned hosiery was a complicated mixture of ingredients. These included zinc oxide and titanium dioxide for an even covering, mixed with iron oxides or other dyes to provide colour, as well as talc to create a the illusion of the sheen of a silk stocking. Glycerine or sorbitol was added to prevent peeling and an adhesive such as casein, a protein derived from cows' milk, or latex, helped the mixture stick to the leg. All this was combined with alcohol to speed up the drying process and prevent smudging or the accidental transference of the product onto clothing or furniture; a tricky business all round.

Cosmetics at the Front

It is distressing to note the case of one World War I soldier who was found to have in his possession at the front a powder puff, which apparently he used or intended to use to tint his cheeks in order that his pallor should not give away just how frightened he was. Aside from the scarcity of cosmetics during World War II and the pressure on women to look good for the war effort, by a twist of fate make-up had another key role to play, this time in respect of men returning from fighting at the front. *Pathfinder News Magazine* ran an item in 1944 under the heading 'Greyed by Battle'.

The article describes how young soldiers in their thousands, serving in the war in Europe and the Pacific, had literally gone grey overnight on account of the trauma of battle. The article goes on to say that base hospitals and rehab centres were asking for hair dyes for these soldiers, who didn't want to return home unless their hair looked their own natural colour. An American manufacture in Stanford Connecticut supplied hair dye free to all soldiers who wanted to cover grey before returning home.

Cosmetic Companies

Many cosmetic companies whose names are very familiar to us today began in very small ways selling perhaps only one product, or specialising in a small range of cosmetics designed to correct or enhance a particular feature; lips, eyes or skin. When Estee Lauder was formed in 1943, it only manufactured six products. Revlon, founded in 1932, originally specialised in nail polish but expanded into lipsticks. Charles of the Ritz sold the first blended powders, made up at point of sale to suit the individual. Although we are used to the idea of individually mixed make-up today, powder bars that offered this service in the 1930s were a novelty. This was a tricky process to get right, given the effects of moving in and out of artificial and natural light. The product was not only made to order but gift wrapped and pretty packaging always appeals to buyers. The sometimes bitter rivalry between cosmetic giants Elizabeth Arden and Helena Rubenstein is well known. Arden (born Florence Nightingale Graham), the youngest daughter of a Scots immigrant and grocer shop owner living in Ontario, sought her fortune in New York, taking her new name from a book she had enjoyed entitled *Elizabeth and her German garden* by Von Arnem. Having opened her Fifth Avenue salon in 1910, Arden, a keen racing fan, used her commercially successful Arden Eight Hour Cream not only for female clients but also on her horses. Rubenstein, a Polish businesswoman and philanthropist whose beginnings were humble, had made her own porcelain looks and strong character work for her, opening her first salon in 1902. In 1914, T. I. Williams set up his company Maybelline, naming it after his sister whom he had observed putting petroleum jelly on her lashes. A few companies initially traded under a different name. L'Oreal founded in 1907 by Eugene Shueller, was originally called the French Harmless Hair Colouring Company and developed the first commercially available hair dye. Cover Girl, a small company at its foundation in 1960, became a big player in the cosmetic market challenging the likes of Revlon and others. Cover Girl made modelling more glamorous and introduced make-up as a self-service item. No need to approach someone at a shop counter. Just pick some products and pay at the desk.

Advertising

In the early part of the twentieth century, advertising of cosmetics was still limited. Many people continued to disapprove of make-up, leading clients to enter cosmetic establishments by a back door. Small, unobtrusive advertisements for make-up in newspapers were the norm. However in 1903, *Vogue* carried its first cosmetic advertisement and started including advice on how to apply make-up within its pages. In 1933, the first advertisement for make-up was broadcast on radio. During the '30s advertising for beauty products became more extensive, glossy and even adventurous. Elizabeth Arden even ran an interactive advertisement in 1939 with a wheel to turn to select the right colour of foundation for you. The American make-up mogul Richard Hudnut made sure his sales staff could show women how to apply his products correctly. Hudnut started out selling perfume but expanded into a wide range of creams, powders, rouges and lipsticks. He also saw the advantages attractive packaging and how it could boost sales.

The advertising of cosmetic products burgeoned after World War II though in the first few years ladies magazines did veer away from advertising as rationing was still in force and the 'make do and mend' mentality took a while to dissipate. Following the war women, it seems, had never had it so good in terms of the availability, the variety and the range of prices for cosmetics. American television tried out a new form of advertising, which was to prove highly successful. A popular American television quiz show called *The 64,000 Dollar Question,* which first appeared on air in 1955, was sponsored by make-up manufacturer Revlon. The company used the show as a vehicle for selling their wares, especially their lipstick. As an advertising medium, this was so successful that once a new shade of Revlon lipstick was seen on screen, it could easily be sold out in the shops a matter of days. Although not direct advertising in the same way, in the 1990s, television research that appeared to scientifically back up the claims made about Boots No 7 Protect and Perfect Anti-Wrinkle Serum produced a shopping frenzy and a run on Boots stores the next day. The desire for the preservation of youth had shown no signs of flagging and advertising, whether on television, radio, in newspaper or magazines proved its worth.

Shopping for Make-up

The secret of the Perfect Complexion of noted beauties of the day is disclosed; and the Remarkable Preparations which have produced and retained these Extraordinary Results at last obtainable by the General Public, although for years they have been exclusively supplied by a Specialist solely to her private patients.

Cyclax advertisement, 1907

Beauty secrets were no longer quite so secret. Selfridges opened its doors in 1909. Cosmetics were on open sale. Even shops in provincial towns sold the latest in make-up products. The American beauty line Dubarry, named after Comtesse Jeanne du Barry (1743–1793), the mistress of Louis XV of France, was developed by American businessman Richard Hudnut. His range included face powder (in two sizes) lipstick, rouge, eye shadow and mascara. Dubarry products were hugely successful and could be bought not only in the big cities but in the smaller towns in Britain, including the county town of Bathgate just outside Edinburgh. Hudnut's lipstick was on sale at the provincial chemist there for 3s 6d, and rouge for 1s 9d. For those who could not get to the shops or who were in search of a particular product not available locally, many companies still offered a mail order service – even posting quite sizeable free samples straight to the door to entice women to buy their product on a regular basis.

Aside from shopping either in large department stores, smaller outlets or perhaps buying by mail order, the customer might also have the option of buying from door-to-door salesmen and women. This method of selling beauty products took hold from the very beginning of the twentieth century. The cosmetic company Avon had specialised in this method of selling in Britain since the end of the nineteenth century. Other door-to-door sales cosmetics sellers include Annie Turnbo, a black businesswoman who began selling hair treatments on the doorstep in America at the turn of the century. Sarah McWilliams also marketed a hair grower in the same way. And other door-to-door options, Mary Kay Cosmetics, a company formed in 1963, remains a popular brand while Avon has displayed remarkable longevity and is still a household name. Cosmetics had moved quite literally out of the closet and into full public view.

Tanning: A New Trend

Dissolve the tragacanth with enough rose water to form thin mucilage. Crush the strawberries; mix and stir them up with a sufficient quantity of rose water to form a half liquid paste ; add the tragacanth and the violet powder; apply the paste to the face at night and wash off next morning with tepid water. It is said that this operation repeated for three successive nights will remove all sunburn and tan.

Harriet Hubbard Ayer

At the turn of the century, Harriet Hubbard Ayer's strawberry paste was being marketed not only as a way of refreshing the complexion and perfuming the skin but also to rid oneself of any evidence of exposure to the sun. However by the 1920s, Riviera holidays in the South of France had become popular for the wealthy and fashions began to change, helped no doubt by one notable figure. The fashion icon Coco Chanel was photographed sporting a deep tan aboard the Duke of Westminster's yacht. Her friend Prince Louise de Faucigny-Lucigne quipped 'I think she [Coco] invented sunbathing. At that time she invented everything.' Alpine ski holidays, which meant exposure to the sun, were also popular with the smart set. The ability to afford a foreign holiday, to lie in the sun as a lady or gentleman of leisure, even if only for a couple of weeks in the year, smacked of wealth and status; the tan was visible proof of that. For those who could not afford the holiday, the sun kissed look could be acquired without the expense of a trip abroad by using saffron, for instance, to dye the skin. However, according to one London newspaper in 1924, 'Parisiennes are forsaking cosmetics owing to male preference for the unadorned complexions which have become popular during seaside and alpine holidays'. Darker complexions in fashion due to the popularity of the tan called for paler lipsticks as a contrast. In 1956 the trade magazine *Chemist and Druggist* advertised the following product, which indicates that make-up companies were rethinking and redesigning their products to match the now fashionable tan; 'For summer make-up Elizabeth Arden ... are issuing to meet the fashion for pale lipsticks contrasting with deeper complexion tones a new lipstick: "Summertime".' Self-tanning began in 1960 using a DHA sugarcane derivative, which stains the outer layers of skin. The exposure of more of the skin to view also prompted widespread advertising of hair removers too.

The Safety of Cosmetics: The Unpleasant and the Downright Dangerous

Fish scales to add shimmer to lipstick and parts of placenta added to the skin creams may seem a little distasteful. However scandals over rather more dangerous substances in modern day cosmetics still crop up. Despite concerns about safety, harmful lead has been found in some lipsticks. Belladonna is still used to create that wide-eyed effect and parabens have been added to cosmetics as preservatives since 1927. Although the latter prevents products becoming infected with harmful bacteria, some people believe these chemicals carry a risk themselves. Those in the medical profession began to express concern that cosmetics were not classified under the Medicines Act, given the not only the ingredients they contained but also on account of the claims that were made for some products.

Mascara for colouring lashes and brows was very much a twentieth century invention and to begin with, serious mistakes were made in terms of the production and composition of this new product. In the 1930s an eye lash dye marketed under the name Lash Lure, and containing the dangerous chemical p-phenylenediamine, a coal tar derivative originally used in the hairdressing industry, caused much misery to many women. This was one of the so-called eye lash beautifiers of which there were a number on the market at the time, which were not safe. Socialite Miss Norris had suffered from the agonies caused by Lash Lure, which destroyed her corneas and eventually rendered her blind. Her case was highlighted in a newsreel produced by Paramount Pictures, who were in the forefront of seeking greater control over the cosmetics industry. In 1933, The American Food and Drugs Agency highlighted the dangers of Lash Lure and other similar products again at the Chicago World Fair with graphic 'before and after' photographs of Miss Norris, who was far from being the only person to suffer but was one of the most severe cases. The display attracted the attention of the first lady Eleanor Roosevelt and in 1938, the Federal Drugs Agency in America gained the power to act against Lash Lure and other American cosmetic manufacturers whose products had done such harm. By this time, sixteen women had lost their sight and one woman had died as a result of using this beauty product. Until 1938, despite the horrors inflicted on individuals who had used Lash Lure and other deadly products, there was no legal right to redress or to stop these being produced.

Radium Glow

In the middle of the twentieth century, one could literally radiate youth and beauty according to advertisements for radium creams, which were selling in the best and most fashionable shops on London and Paris. In fact, there was quite a craze for radium products of all sorts. This was something that was added to everything from chocolate to underwear as well as cosmetics and sold to unwitting consumers. One company Radior produced a wide range of cosmetic products based on the supposed benefits of radium that included night creams, hair tonics and face powders. In 1918, Radior promoted their products promising that, 'an overflowing fountain of youth has at last been found in the energy rays of radium ... radium rays revitalize and energise all living tissue'. As a result of using products based on radium women literally glowed in the dark. And this included women who worked in the factories that made these products as well as those who actually wore make-up based on radium. Cases of radium sickness and illnesses that developed years later were the result.

Mercolised Wax, 'the Modern Skin Beautifier'

Advertised as a means of improving one's complexion by removing any pigmentation defects, and even signs of the diseases like syphilis, while at the same time lightening the skin 'without the use of cosmetics' mercolised wax was, an effect, a chemical peel. Applied at night to the face and washed off in the morning, the wax removed dead skin. *The Scotsman* newspaper carried this short piece in 1914, entitled 'To Renew Complexions without Cosmetics':

> If the excessive user of cosmetics only knew the impression her artificiality really makes upon others she would quickly seek the means of gaining a natural complexion. Let her acquire the mercolised wax habit discarding make-up entirely and she will soon have the kind of complexion that women envy and men admire. It is so easy to get a little mercolised wax from the chemist and use it nightly like cold cream washing it off in the morning. Gradually the lifeless soiled outer cuticle peels off in tiny invisible flakes and in a week or so you have a brand new complexion clear, soft, velvety and of girlish colour and texture. The treatment is so simple, harmless and marvellously effective the wonder is that every woman whose skin is withered and discoursed has not already adopted it.

Advertisements claimed that mercolised wax was 'guaranteed not to contain any form of mercury'. However, as mercury was one of its main ingredients this was far from the truth. An application of mercolised wax was not a safe procedure at all. Indeed, only a year after its appearance on the market in 1911 the American Medical Association had stated that the stuff 'is a caustic poison and in the interests of the public safety the law should require that it be held such'. While its use could, in the short term, reduce pigmentation and lighten the skin, the long-term effects of using it could be fatal. Legal restrictions on the use of mercury in make-up were not applied in Europe and the United States until the 1970s. An advertisement for Rowland's Kalydor published in newspapers and magazines at the beginning of the twentieth century, a face product that promised a pale and blemish-free complexion, also makes clear that the removal of freckles remained desirable. It is unclear what this mixture sold in bottles actual consisted of, though it was claimed that it was made 'for the most part from eastern balsamic exotics'. We are none the wiser.

The Twentieth Century: The Later Years

The 1940s and '50s saw a demand for easily portable cosmetics, such as powder compacts. The cosy appeal of the girl next-door look was popularised by actresses such as Doris Day in the films of the day. This trend was reflected in understated make-up, with a little rouge that gave a healthy glow. The '70s and '80s saw a brief resurgence in very elaborate make-up, modelled on some of the music bands that used it as part of their act at the time; fans copied their style. An interest in all things Gothic led to young people using black make-up as a mark of belonging to that particular grouping. In contrast, Biba's extreme make-up was highly colourful. Nail polish in a huge range of colours became the height of fashion thanks to technology originally used to develop paints for the car industry.

There was not only a move towards regulation, and therefore greater safety of cosmetic products, but also a forceful, sometimes violent, movement against testing cosmetics on animals emerged. Ethics became the new watchword. Begun as a cottage industry by its founder Anita Roddick, The Body Shop based it products on ethically sourced natural ingredients from around the world. In 1988 *The Times* stated that, 'demand for the Body Shop's no hype cosmetics is growing so fast that the group is having to control its outlets to maintain standards at this point'. Roddick's British market was now fully developed but there were still only a few outlets that sold her products in Europe, with no shops in the United States. Expansion continued and other companies marketing safe and ethically sources make-up followed. Inventively, cosmetics in the latter twenty years of the twentieth century managed to combine individualism with belonging; one could express oneself through make-up as well as indicate your allegiance to a particular social group linked by a taste in music, fashion and ideology.

Popular Products

Brylcreem, first manufactured by County Chemicals in Birmingham in 1928, is a more modern version of the hair pomade. A mixture of mineral oils and beeswax, this product was intended to add gloss to the hair and to keep the style in place. In the '30s and '40s, a well-groomed appearance was still important, an indication perhaps not so much about class but about one's organised lifestyle and overall morality. The packaging may have been fairly plain and did not change much over the years, but the manufacturers of Brylcreem did see the importance of advertising their brand successfully. In Britain, they did so using a half-page newspaper advert, using the popular sport of cricket as its medium to advertise the new product. The company supported its sellers with attractive display items so that they could show off their wares to best effect in their shop windows or on shelf displays. After World War II, however, men out of service and back on Civvy Street took the opportunity to grow their hair a little longer, which meant there was less demand for this sort of cosmetic product. Although it would never be as ubiquitous as it was before World War II, by using David Beckham as their 'face' on advertisements in the 1990s, the manufacturers did introduce their product to a whole new generation. Brylcreem is still available and its familiar packaging remains unchanged.

Scented face powders that not only smelled good but took away any shine from the nose or chin became popular in the 1920s. The shine or glimmer so much admired in ancient times was no longer appreciated. Lillie Powder was named after Lillie Langtry, the famous musical star and mistress of King Edward VII. The powder consisted of talcum powder stained with carmine and sienna, mixed with melted lanolin, and scented with violet perfume, producing a tinted and scented face powder.

In the 1920s well-to-do ladies covered their faces with veils in the daytime. This no doubt protected their faces from the elements but may also have concealed a poor complexion. The American company producing this cream stated in their advertisements,

> You don't need to wear a veil. The soft smooth picture of healthy skin which nature gives to all children is yours by right and every girl or woman can if she will retain or regain the perfect pretty complexion of childhood simply by a few moments of massage with Pompeian Massage Cream.

There were a number of products in the Pompeian range including massage cream, day cream and night cream. All recalled the heady days of ancient Rome. The advertisements for the preparations promised a success in love. 'Make cupid a caller' was the headline in one advertisement:

> He is waiting round the corner of life there – ready to bring you joy and happiness. If only the women uses the cream to make such a difference in herself she will become a woman that men must love.

On the one hand, this is Mills & Boon stuff, but it also puts the onus on the woman in the most patronising way, casting her as siren with powers that bewitch men. She is everything, and it is her fault if she is not using their cream.

Telling Twentieth-Century Advertising Slogans

Don't envy Beauty: Use Pompeian, Pompeian Face Cream (1910s)
You too can have eyes that charm!: Eye shadow by Maybelline (1920s)

Paris knows the way to keep that school girl complexion: Palmolive soap (1930s)

Choose your make-up by the colour of your eyes: Richard Hudnut's Eye Matched Make-up (1930s)

Help yourself to love romance and popularity with a pretty brighter looking skin: Sweet Georgia Brown Bleach cream. (1940s)

For dream hands cream your hands: Madeleine Carroll Pacquin's Hand Cream (1940s)

I never dreamed I'd look this young at my age: Revenescence Face Cream by Charles of the Ritz (1950)

She never looks made-up ... her skin glows with the softness of candlelight: Touch n Glow by Revlon (1950s)

Irresistible: It's easy to be a glamour girl: Irresistible range (1950s)

Luscious licks of bare frosty colour that looks like you do soaking wet: lipstick by Clairol (1960s)

Beautifully bared. Softer than yesterday: Ultralucent make-up by Max Factor (1960s)

At last! A Cover Girl Complexion so natural you can't believe it's not make-up: Noxzema Medicated Make-up by Cover Girl (1960s)

A new look in faces –smooth mysterious lustrous to make yesterday's make-up seem dated: New Illusion Foundation by Elizabeth Arden (1960s)

She couldn't fix a proper cup of tea. She even beat him at darts. But he loved her madly because of her English Eyes: Eye shadow by Yardley of London (1970s)

Why should it just be nature that changes her face for Autumn?: Autumn make-up range by Mary Quant (1970s)

Lesson number one in social graces. Never be offensive: Right Guard deodorant for men (1980s)

By the time you've finished your left foot your right foot will ready to go: Cutex Color Quick Polish – Colorful Toe Nails (1990s).

9

THE TWENTY-FIRST CENTURY:
MAKING UP IN PUBLIC WITH MAKE-UP FROM THE PAST

The best thing is to look natural, but it takes make-up to look natural.

Calvin Klein, fashion designer

While ethical and, to a large extent, safety considerations in respect of cosmetics are modern concerns, there are the many other ideas associated with owning, applying or wearing make-up that are not linked to a particular era and that occur again and again throughout history. Chief among these are standards of feminine beauty, the physical appearance of good health, appropriate etiquette (especially in public), the expression of wealth, an indication of social status, a gender distinction, an element of disguise, a striving for perfection, the meaning of colour, the preservation of youth, the rhetorical nature versus artifice debate, the essentials of fashion and the mark of ethnicity: a long list indeed.

Let us take a look at the concept of beauty in the first instance. Fashions may have come and gone but some of the standard elements of Western beauty have remained static; in particular, well-groomed hair (especially the appreciation of blonde hair) and sparkling bright eyes are still considered attractive. However, there are differences. While some result from developments in technology (for example, the proliferation of nail varnish or waterproof cosmetics) others do not exclude or detract from more traditional and longstanding elements of perfect beauty. For example the popularity of a tan, for women at least, is one major break with the past but although the sun-kissed look is fashionable, a pale complexion remains a feature to be appreciated too. In addition, while the trend towards conforming to the current ideal (or following fashion, if you like) still exists, twenty-first century society appears far more accepting of individual expression and therefore extremes, for example, hair dyed an unnatural pink, blue or green is not uncommon.

What about health and wellbeing? In 1950, a report from The American Society of Chemists quoted in the British Press stated that: 'Cosmetics in the future will increasingly assume the function of preventative medicine in addition to their present aim of beautifying the human body'. Perhaps these chemists were forgetting that cosmetics had long found common ground with medicines from ancient times. However, it is true to say that in this, the twenty first century, we have seen a return to crediting make-up with potential benefits that may be more than skin deep. The word 'cosmeceutical', meaning 'a cosmetic product which contains active ingredients that have a beneficial effect on the user's body', coined at the end of the twentieth century, is now becoming more widely used and ironically, cosmetics that have been around for many hundreds if not thousands of years fit the definition: kohl, rosewater, frankincense and myrrh, to name but a few. There are other benefits that have come about as a result of cosmetics reclaiming association with medicines too, not least the fact that they have been proven to make women, in particular, feel better. Cancer patents in hospital may be offered make-up to help give them confidence in their appearance when undergoing treatment, nursing homes for the elderly aim to provide regular hair care services for their residents. For women and men disfigured by an accident, cosmetics can disguise the damage.

On a less positive note, the 'medicinal' properties of make-up are sometimes sold to us in adverts using pseudo-scientific words and making enticing claims that cannot be proven. This is particularly true of the market in anti-aging creams. Advanced anti-aging creams claim to boost gene activity and stimulate protein production, helping us look younger than we are. Western society has always equated youth with beauty and women will pay high prices for creams that seem to offer the promise to eternal youth.

Aside from expensive face creams with unproven benefits, there are potentially dangerous beauty products on the market too. Despite legislation to prevent harmful cosmetics being manufactured, some of the dangerous ingredients used in the past are still with us in the present. A report into lipsticks in 2007, undertaken by the an American research group called The Campaign for Safer Cosmetics, found that sixty per cent of lipsticks still contained small amounts of lead. This was especially the case with regard to red lipstick. Furthermore, while a tan may be an indication of health and a good level of fitness, the tanning process itself can be detrimental to one's wellbeing. Health scares surrounding tanning, natural or otherwise, have led to a resurgence of the pale and interesting look, although acquiring a fair complexion through the use of make-up can have its dangers too. Whitening salons are commonplace in towns and cities in China, where laser techniques are used to whiten the skin to make Asian men and women look more European; in that part of the world, pale skin is still taken as an indication of affluence. However, this is an expensive procedure so many choose to buy lightening creams at beauty counters. Even some of the authorised brands on sale contain toxic ingredients, such as mercury. There is the matter of gender to consider too.

In Europe, make-up for men is again becoming more mainstream with a wide range of products, especially for skin care, readily available on the shelves of both larger and smaller shops. Mac cosmetics recently launched a uni-sex make-up range advertised on YouTube using male models. However, the use of make-up by men in today's world still has a long way to go to reach the levels of use this achieved in the seventeenth and eighteenth centuries.

There has been one very significant change over the last few years and that is the fact that the process of applying one's make-up has gone from being a very private ritual to an increasingly public event. Nail bars and eye brow shaping salons have sprung up in the most public of places, not only inside shops but in the concourses of major shopping centres. The public face of make-up is a far cry from the application of cosmetics behind closed doors that was normal practice even in the latter part of the twentieth century. Consider the argument against this, presented in an article in *The Telegraph* online in May 2011: 'Why bother with the whole charade if you're going to let the outside world into every step of the process? What is the point of erecting a formal façade ... if you're publicly admitting the fraudulence of it all?' Not only does the whole debate around nature and artifice raise its head again, but the secrets and the mystique surrounding cosmetics kept for hundreds of years are lost and there is, it seems to me, some regret in that. However, the idea of owning, wearing and flaunting cosmetics as a symbol of wealth and status has not gone away. In August 2015 *The Times* newspaper ran an article commenting on the large number of expensive face creams on the market, costing around the £500 mark. The headline reads, 'Impress by having a jar of ... on the shelf in your bathroom, Expensive face creams: a must-have status item.' The pressure on women to buy the best they can afford, and to spend vast sums of money on something that is not proven to work, is immense. This is little different from the pressures on the ladies who ran up large bills at Madame Rachel's exotic cosmetic salon in Bond Street in the nineteenth century..

While the ability to purchase exclusive skin creams and other make-up items may tell us something about the individual, the sales of cosmetics *per se* have been discovered to be an accurate gauge of the state of the economy in general. Basically, in a recession sales of red lipstick go up but when the financial situation improves nude lipstick shades are more popular. Although economists were aware of this trend during the Great Depression of the 1930s, it was only given the name the Lipstick Index by Leonard Lauder, the chairman of the cosmetics company Estee Lauder, in 2001. The reasoning behind this phenomenon has been interpreted thus – red lipstick represents the defiant struggle to find optimism in time of crisis but when there is no need to stand out in this way, nude shades become fashionable again.

Just as it does in respect of many things, the past informs the future as far as cosmetics are concerned. Cosmetic companies, for example L'Oreal and Olay, have spent time, money, and effort researching cosmetics used in the past in the belief that what can be learned from this can make a worthwhile contribution to the design and manufacture of cosmetics in the future. Their faith seems well founded. For example, remember the ingredients in the Roman poet Ovid's face pack recipes. Recent research has found that those lupin seeds have a proven positive effective on the skin. Frankincense is another commodity valued in antiquity. The extract from oil of frankincense is now believed to have an anti-aging effect too. Alpha Hydroxy Acid (AHA), basically a chemical peel derived from natural products including fruit and milk, may reduce wrinkles. Cleopatra, when bathing in milk, was on to a good thing even though she did not, in scientific terms, know why. Other cosmetics with a long history that are still used today include kaolin or china clay, used as foundation by the Romans. This is a common ingredient in modern powdered make-up.

Cinnamon is still used in toothpaste and men's cosmetics. Aloe and almond oil are popular in modern skin creams for their soothing qualities. Lanolin, naturally developed by sheep to keep their skin and wool in good condition, continues to be mostly beneficial with little toxicity for most humans. Other uses have been found for some age-old cosmetic ingredients. For example, laurel leaves are no longer chewed to freshen breath but are thought beneficial as an ingredient in anti-dandruff shampoos. Barley and bran are, as they always have been, effective exfoliators though both now double as effective ingredients in shampoos. Tattoos are very fashionable for both men and women in modern society, stemming perhaps from a basic need in man to decorate himself. Reality and the rhetoric, that is nature and artifice, co-exist in any given era. The women in the fashion pages, airbrushed and Photoshopped, are no more an achievable representation of our selves than the idealised women described in literature and depicted in the artwork of the past. However, the use of foundation, powder, breath fresheners, hair dyes, rouge and other beauty products is not simply a fashionable element of dress but a feature of appearance underpinned by ideas of beauty, contemporary etiquette, social status, health and wellbeing, wealth and gender and, as such, an effective means of understanding our past – and our present.

GLOSSARY OF COSMETIC INGREDIENTS

Alabaster: Fine grained white or light coloured translucent gypsum, often streaked or mottled. Soft and easily carved.

Alkanet: A European plant, *Alkania tinctoria*, the root of this plant, or a dye prepared from it. Also called bugloss.

Almond oil: Oil extracted from almonds, rich in vitamin E, the tree is native to Middle East, Indian subcontinent and North Africa.

Aloe: African plant with long, fleshy spiny-edged leaves.

Alum: Any double sulphate of a monovalent metal or radical (such as sodium, potassium, or ammonium) and a trivalent metal (such as aluminium or iron).

Ammoniac: Strong-smelling gum resin from the stems of a plant, *Dorema ammoniacum*, of North Africa. This is also known gum ammoniac.

Angelica: Any plant of the genus Angelica. Mostly Eurasian in distribution, they are tall, perennial herbs with divided leaves and clusters of white or greenish flowers.

Antimony: Metallic element. the most common form of this is a hard, extremely brittle, lustrous, silver-white, crystalline material.

Arsenic: The proper name for this is arsenic trioxide: it is a highly poisonous white powdery substance.

Azurite: Azure-blue vitreous mineral of basic copper carbonate.

Balsam: An umbrella term for aromatic resins obtained from a variety of different trees and shrubs.

Beeswax: the yellowish to dark brown wax secreted by the honey bee for making honeycombs.

Belladonna: A poisonous plant with purple flowers also known as deadly nightshade.

Benzoin: A fragrant gum resin obtained from trees of the genus styrax.

Bisort: Any of several plants of the genus Polygonum, especially a Eurasian plant, *P. Bistorta*, having pointed clusters of small, pinkish flowers. Also called snakeroot or snakeweed.

Bitumen: Any of various mixtures of hydrocarbons, occurring naturally or obtained by distillation from coal or petroleum, found in asphalt or tar.

Borage: A flowering herb.

Borax: Hydrous sodium borate, a crystalline compound found on the shores of hot springs and in the dry beds of salt lakes in arid regions.

Brazilwood: The red wood of any of several tropical trees of the genus Caesalpina.

Brimstone: Old name for sulphur. This is a pale yellow non-metallic element that occurs **naturally.**

Camphor: – A volatile crystalline compound obtained from camphor tree wood.

Carmine: A crimson pigment derived from cochineal. *see* Cochineal.

Carob: An evergreen tree of the Mediterranean region, having compound leaves. The pods are edible.

Ceruse: White lead, a heavy white poisonous compound of basic lead carbonate, lead silicate or lead sulphate.

Chypre: A perfume or group of perfumes named after the island of Cyprus, of which sandalwood is an important ingredient.

Cinnabar: Mercuric sulphide. It is deposited in veins and impregnations near recent volcanic rocks and hot springs. The mineral itself is used as a red pigment, commonly known as 'vermilion'.

Cochineal: A tropical American scale insect, that feeds on certain types of cacti. A brilliant red dye is made by drying and pulverising the bodies of the female. *see* Carmine.

Dragon's blood: A red gum that exudes from the fruit of some palms and from the dragon tree that originates in the Canary Isles.

Frankincense: Resin of various African and Asian trees of the genus Boswellia.

Galena: Chief ore of lead, consisting of lead sulphide. It is lead-grey in colour and has a high metallic lustre.

Gall Nuts: A plant gall having a rounded form suggestive of a nut being an abnormal swelling of plant tissue, caused by insects, micro-organisms or external injury.

Glycerine: A colourless sweet sticky liquid formed as a by-product of soap making.

Gum Arabic: A gum exuded by various African trees of the genus Acacia,. This is also called acacia.

Gypsum: A hydrated form of the white crystalline sold calcium sulphate.

Hartshorn: a liquid ammonia derived from the horns of male deer.

Haematite: A principle ore of iron, consisting mainly of iron oxide. It occurs as specular haematite (dark, metallic lustre), kidney ore (reddish radiating fibres terminating in smooth, rounded surfaces) and as a red earthy deposit.

Henbane: A poisonous plant native to the Mediterranean region with unpleasant odour.

Henna: A tree or shrub, *Lawsonia inernis,* of Asia and northern Africa, having fragrant white or reddish flowers. (b) A reddish powder obtained from the leaves of this plant.

Honey: Sweet syrup produced by honey bees from the nectar of flowers. It is stored in honeycombs and made in excess of their needs as food for the winter. Honey comprises various sugars, mainly laevulose and dextrose, with enzymes, colouring matter, acids and pollen grain. It has anti-bacterial properties.

Hydrochloric acid: a solution of Hydrogen chloride (colourless gas) mixed with water

Kaolin: A fine white to yellowish or grey clay, mostly kaolinite, also known as china clay or porcelain clay.

Kohl: Powdered antimony sulphide.

Lac: A resin secreted by the lac insect.

Lanolin: Sticky, purified wax obtained from sheep's wool.

Lapis lazuli: Rock containing the blue mineral lazurite. It is found in Afghanistan, Siberia, Iran and Chile.

Lepidocrocite, also called esmeraldite or hydrohematite: This is an iron oxide-hydroxide mineral. *Lepidocrocite* has crystal structure, a lustre and a yellow-brown streak. It is most often found growing inside quartz. It forms when iron-bearing minerals are exposed to oxidation and / or weathering. The colouring of lepidocrocite usually ranges from red to dark red to reddish brown often dependent upon the quartz where it takes up residence. For example, when this mineral is found inside amethyst, its colouring is generally more purplish-red.

Litharge: A red crystalline form of lead monoxide

Lye: A strong alkaline solution

Malachite: Common copper ore, basic copper carbonate. Green in colour

Mallow: Any flowering plant of the genus Malvaceae.

Mastic: The aromatic resin of the mastic tree, *Pistacin lentisus*. Originally a sap, mastic is sun-dried into pieces of brittle, translucent resin.

Mercury, also called 'quicksilver': A silvery-white poisonous metallic element, liquid at room temperature.

Mother of Pearl: The smooth, lustrous lining in the shells of certain molluscs – for example pearl oysters, abalones and mussels. Mother of pearl consists of calcium carbonate.

Musk: A greasy secretion with a powerful odour, produced in a glandular sac beneath the skin of the abdomen of the male musk deer, and any similar secretion of certain other vertebrates, such as the civet and otter, also synthetic chemical resembling same.

Myrrh: An aromatic gum resin obtained from several trees and plants of the genus Commiphora, that grow India, Arabia and eastern Africa.

Natron: A mineral form of hydrous sodium carbonate, often found crystallised with other salts.

Ochre: Any of several earthy mineral oxides of iron mingled with various amounts of clay and sand, occurring in yellow, brown or red.

Oil of turps or turpentine: Refined turpentine, a thin volatile essential oil, consisting of a mixture of terpenes, obtained by steam distillation or other means from the wood or the exudate of various pine trees.

Orpiment: A mineral, arsenic trisulphide, used as lemon yellow pigment.

Orris root: The fragrant root of the orris, any of several species of iris.

Potassium Permanganate: A purple crystalline solid.

Pyrite, also called fool's gold or iron pyrites: A yellow to brown, widely occurring mineral sulphide, used as an iron ore and to produce sulphur dioxide for sulphuric acid.

Quicklime: Calcium oxide. This substance is so called because it is the first substance produced by heating limestone.

Quicksilver: *see* Mercury.

Radish: Any of various plants of the genus Raphanus, especially *R. sativus,* having a thickened edible root. Also the root itself.

Rosemary: An aromatic, evergreen shrub, native to southern Europe but widely cultivated, having light blue flowers and greyish-green leaves.

Red Ochre: *see* Ochre.

Saffron: Orange flavouring and colouring from the dried stigmas of the crocus flower.

Sandalwood: Scented red wood of the sandal tree.

Spermaceti: Glistening wax-like substance, not true oil, contained in the cells of the huge, almost rectangular 'case' in the head of the sperm whale, amounting to about 2.8 tonnes. It rapidly changes in density with variations in temperature.

Styrax (or storax): A tree resin

Sulphur: *see* Brimstone.

Tannin: a complex group of organic compounds found in tree bark or in oak galls.

Tartar: A reddish acid compound, chiefly potassium bitartrate, found in the juice of grapes and deposited on the sides of casks during wine-making.

Terebinth: A small southern European tree

Titanium oxide: A metallic naturally occurring white pigment

Vermilion: *see* Cinnabar.

White lead: *see* Ceruse.

Wormwood: Any of several aromatic plants of the genus Artemisia, especially *A. absinthium,* native to Europe.

Yellow ochre: *see* Ochre

Zinc Oxide: White metallic element.

SELECT BIBLIOGRAPHY

General

Winter, Ruth M. S., *A Consumers Dictionary of Cosmetic Ingredients* (New York: Random House Publishing, 2005)

Sherrow, Victoria, *For Appearance' Sake: The Historical Encyclopaedia of Good Looks, Beauty and Grooming* (Connecticut: Oryx Press, 2001)

Ancient World

Stewart, Susan, *Cosmetics and Perfumes in the Roman World* (Stroud: Tempus, 2007)

Johnson, Marguerite, *Ovid on Cosmetics: Medicamina Faciei Femineae and Related Texts* (London: Bloomsbury Academic, 2016)

The Middle Ages

Green, Monica, *The Trotula: An English Translation of the Medieval Companion of Women's Medicine* (Philadelphia: University of Pennsylvania Press, 2002)

Fifteenth and Sixteenth Centuries

Bell, Rudolph, M., *How to do it: Guides to Good Living for Renaissance Italians* (Chicago and London: University of Chicago Press, 1999)

Fornaciai, Valentina, *Toilet Perfumes and Make-up at the Medici Court: Pharmaceutical Recipe Books, Florentine Collection and Medici Milieu Uncovered* (Livorno: Sillabe, 2007)

Karim-Cooper, Farah, *Cosmetics in Shakespearean and Renaissance Drama* (Edinburgh: Edinburgh University Press, 2012)

Wheeler, Jo, and Temple, Katy, *Renaissance Secrets, Recipes and Formulas* (London: V&A Publishing, 2009)

Seventeenth Century

Greig, Hannah, Hamlett, Jane and Hannan, Leon (eds), *Gender and Material Culture in Britain since 1600* (London: Palgrave, 2016)

Read, Sara, *Maids, Wives, Widows: Exploring Early Modern Women's Lives 1540–1740* (Barnsley: Pen and Sword History, 2015)

Eighteenth Century

Bashor, Will, *Marie Antoinette's Head: The Royal Hairdresser, The Queen and The Revolution* (Connecticut: Rowman and Littlefield, 2015)

Nineteenth Century

Kloester, Jennifer, *Georgette Heyer's Regency World* (London: Arrow Books, 2005)

Rappaport, Helen, *Beautiful for Ever: Madame Rachel of Bond Street – Cosmetician, Con-Artist and Blackmailer* (London: Vintage Books, 2012)

Try it! Buy it! Vintage Adverts (London: The British Library, 2015)

Twentieth Century

Masset, Claire, *Department Stores* (Oxford: Shire Publications, 2010)

ACKNOWLEDGEMENTS

Many thanks to Alicia Shultz of LBCC Historical Apothecary (https://www.etsy.com/ie/shop/LitttleBits) and to Hillary, Curator of The Make-up Museum (http://www.makeupmuseum.org) for supplying a number of the photographs. Grateful thanks to Anna Canning, Lucy Ribchester and Kirsty Stewart for their unfailing encouragement and support with this project.

Thank you too to Amberley Publishing for the opportunity to publish this volume, especially to Shaun Barrington who never sounded harassed despite the avalanche of emails I sent him.

Most of all thank you to my husband for his forbearance throughout and his willingness to proofread.

INDEX